IMG Friendly Obstetrics and Gynecology Residency Programs List

With Comprehensive Match Selection Criteria and Programs Requirements.

By

IMG Guide
and
Applicant Guide

Table of Contents

Introduction

IMG Friendly Obstetrics and Gynecology Residency Programs List With Match Selection Criteria and Programs Requirements.

In Collaboration between the Applicant Guide and the IMG Guide we present to you the most complete and up-to-date IMG friendly Obstetrics and Gynecology residency programs list with full match selection criteria and requirements for these programs. This book is essentially written for international medical graduates seeking residency in the US. The idea of writing this book came from our insight that many IMGs every year don't match because they don't know where to apply. Most of the time, they end applying to programs that don't have IMGs or those that don't match their criteria hence they end losing money with no interviews earned. The information was gathered from program directors, coordinators, chiefs, faculty and residents. It includes Programs names, Programs codes, States, Addresses, Phones, Faxes, Percentage of IMGs in the programs, Minimum USMLE Step 1 and Step 2 Score Requirements, Attempts on any step, CS requirement at time of application, USCE Requirements, Cut-Off time since graduation, Programs offering couple match and Visas Sponsored or accepted.

not affiliated to ECFMG, ERAS, NRMP or USMLE.

Alabama

University of South Alabama Obstetrics and Gynecology Residency Program

Specialty: Obstetrics and Gynecology OB GYN Residency
Program name: University of South Alabama Program
Program code: 220-01-21-020
NRMP Code: 1852220C0
Program type: University-based
State: Alabama
Address: University of South Alabama Medical Center,
　　　　251 Cox St, Mobile, AL 36604
Phone: (251) 415-1557
Fax: (251) 415-1552
Percentage of IMGs in the program: 8%
Minimum USMLE Step 1 Score Requirement: No limits set
Minimum USMLE Step 2 Score Requirement: No limits set
Attempts on any step: Must pass on first attempt
CS required at time of application: Yes as well as ECFMG certificate
USCE Requirement: None
Cut-Off time since graduation: No limits set
Program offers couple match: Yes
Visas Sponsored or accepted: J1 visa

Arizona

Phoenix Integrated Residency Obstetrics and Gynecology Residency Program

Specialty: Obstetrics and Gynecology OB GYN Residency
Program name: Phoenix Integrated Residency Program
Program code: 220-03-21-328
NRMP Code: 1898220C0, 1898220P0
Program type: Community-based university affiliated hospital
State: Arizona
Address: Maricopa Medical Center
2601 E Roosevelt St, Phoenix, AZ 85008
Phone: (602) 344-5084
Fax: (602) 344-5894
Percentage of IMGs in the program: 10%
Minimum USMLE Step 1 Score Requirement: 210
Minimum USMLE Step 2 Score Requirement: 210

Attempts on any step: Must pass maximum on 2nd attempt including CS exam
CS required at time of application: Yes including ECFMG certificate
USCE Requirement: None
Cut-Off time since graduation: No limits set
Program offers couple match: No
Visas Sponsored or accepted: No visa

California

Loma Linda University Obstetrics and Gynecology Residency Program

Specialty: Obstetrics and Gynecology OB GYN Residency
Program name: Loma Linda University Program
Program code: 220-05-21-329
State: California
Address: Loma Linda University Medical Center 11234 Anderson St, Loma Linda, CA

92354
Phone: (909) 651-5534
Fax: (909) 651-5401
Percentage of IMGs in the program: 10%
Minimum USMLE Step 1 Score Requirement:
No limits set
Minimum USMLE Step 2 Score Requirement:
No limits set
Attempts on any step: No limits set
CS required at time of application: No
but PTAL/Status letter is required
USCE Requirement: None
Cut-Off time since graduation: 5 years
Program offers couple match: Yes
Visas Sponsored or accepted: J1 visa

Kern Medical Center Obstetrics and Gynecology Residency Program

Specialty: Obstetrics and Gynecology OB
GYN Residency
Program name: Kern Medical Center
Program
Program code: 220-05-31-027
NRMP Code: 1921220C0
Program type: Community-based
State: California
Address: Kern Medical Center
1700 Mount Vernon Ave,

Bakersfield, CA 93306
Phone: (661) 326-2237
Fax: (661) 326-2235
Percentage of IMGs in the program: 10%
(variable)
**Minimum USMLE Step 1 Score
Requirement:** No limits set
**Minimum USMLE Step 2 Score
Requirement:** No limits set
Attempts on any step: Must pass on first
attempt
CS required at time of application: Yes
including ECFMG certificate as well as
PTAL/Status letter
USCE Requirement: None
Cut-Off time since graduation: No limits
set
Program offers couple match: Yes
Visas Sponsored or accepted: No visa

UCLA Medical Center Obstetrics and Gynecology Residency Program

Specialty: Obstetrics and Gynecology OB GYN
Residency
Program name: UCLA Medical Center Program
Program code: 220-05-31-038

NRMP Code: 1956220P0, 1956220C0
Program type: University-based
State: California
Address: UCLA Medical Center
10833 Le Conte Ave, Los Angeles, CA 90095-1740
Phone: (310) 825-9945
Fax: (310) 206-7186
Percentage of IMGs in the program: 5%
Minimum USMLE Step 1 Score Requirement: No limits set
Minimum USMLE Step 2 Score Requirement: No limits set
Attempts on any step: Must pass maximum from 2nd attempt
CS required at time of application: Yes including ECFMG certificate as well as PTAL/Status letter
USCE Requirement: None
Cut-Off time since graduation: No limits set
Program offers couple match: Yes
Visas Sponsored or accepted: J1 visa

Colorado

University of Colorado Obstetrics and Gynecology Residency Program

Specialty: Obstetrics and Gynecology OB GYN Residency
Program name: University of Colorado Program
Program code: 220-07-31-052
NRMP Code: 1076220P0, 1076220C0
Program type: University-based
State: Colorado
Address: University of Colorado Denver School of Medicine
        12631 E 17th Ave, Aurora, CO 80045
Phone: (303) 724-2052
Fax: (303) 724-2055
Percentage of IMGs in the program: 8%
Minimum USMLE Step 1 Score Requirement: 220
Minimum USMLE Step 2 Score Requirement: 220
Attempts on any step: Must pass on first attempt including CS exam
CS required at time of application: Yes including ECFMG certificate
USCE Requirement: None
Cut-Off time since graduation: No limits set
Program offers couple match: Yes
Visas Sponsored or accepted: J1 visa

Connecticut

Bridgeport Hospital/Yale University Obstetrics and Gynecology Residency Program

Specialty: Obstetrics and Gynecology OB GYN Residency
Program name: Bridgeport Hospital/Yale University Program
Program code: 220-08-11-054
NRMP Code: 1079220C0
Program type: Community-based university affiliated hospital
State: Connecticut
Address: Bridgeport Hospital
            267 Grant St, Bridgeport, CT 06610
Phone: (203) 384-3990
Fax: (203) 384-3715
Percentage of IMGs in the program: 40%
Minimum USMLE Step 1 Score Requirement: No limits set
Minimum USMLE Step 2 Score Requirement: No limits set
Attempts on any step: No limits set
CS required at time of application: No
USCE Requirement: None
Cut-Off time since graduation: No limits set
Program offers couple match: Yes

Visas Sponsored or accepted: J1 visa and H1b visa

Yale-New Haven Medical Center Obstetrics and Gynecology Residency Program

Specialty: Obstetrics and Gynecology OB GYN Residency
Program name: Yale-New Haven Medical Center Program
Program code: 220-08-21-060
NRMP Code: 1089220C0, 1089220P1
Program type: University-based
State: Connecticut
Address: Yale-New Haven Medical Center
          333 Cedar St, New Haven, CT 06520-8063
Phone: (203) 785-4004
Fax: (203) 785-6586
Percentage of IMGs in the program: 0% (Occasional 1)
Minimum USMLE Step 1 Score Requirement: 215
Minimum USMLE Step 2 Score Requirement: No limits set
Attempts on any step: No limits set
CS required at time of application: No
USCE Requirement: Yes 1 month

Cut-Off time since graduation: No limits set
Program offers couple match: Yes
Visas Sponsored or accepted: J1 visa (H1b visa for exceptional candidates)

District of Columbia

Washington Hospital Center Obstetrics and Gynecology Residency Program

Specialty: Obstetrics and Gynecology
Program name: Washington Hospital Center Program
Program code: 220-10-31-067
NRMP Code: 1800220C0
Program type: Community-based University affiliated hospital
State: District of Columbia
Address: Washington Hospital Center
        110 Irving St NW, Washington, DC 20010-2975
Phone: (202) 877-8035
Fax: (202) 877-5435
Percentage of IMGs in the program: 10%
Minimum USMLE Step 1 Score Requirement: No limits set

Minimum USMLE Step 2 Score Requirement:
No limits set
Attempts on any step: No limits set
CS required at time of application: Yes
USCE Requirement: None
Cut-Off time since graduation: No limits set
Program offers couple match: Yes
Visas Sponsored or accepted: J1 visa

George Washington University Obstetrics and Gynecology Residency Program

Specialty: Obstetrics and Gynecology
Program name: George Washington University Program
Program code: 220-10-21-064
State: District of Columbia
Address: George Washington University Medical Center
2150 Pennsylvania Ave NW, Washington, DC 20037
Phone: (202) 741-2532
Fax: (202) 741-2550
Percentage of IMGs in the program: 10%
Minimum USMLE Step 1 Score Requirement:
220

Minimum USMLE Step 2 Score Requirement:
220
Attempts on any step: Must pass on first attempt
CS required at time of application: No
USCE Requirement: None
Cut-Off time since graduation: No limits set
Program offers couple match: Yes
Visas Sponsored or accepted: J1 visa

Florida

Bayfront Medical Center Obstetrics and Gynecology Residency Program

Specialty: Obstetrics and Gynecology
Program name: Bayfront Medical Center Program
Program code: 220-11-11-074
NRMP Code: 1911220C0
Program type: Community-based
State: Florida
Address: Bayfront Health St Petersburg
700 6th St S, St Petersburg, FL 33701
Phone: (727) 893-6917
Fax: (727) 893-6978
Percentage of IMGs in the program: 40%

Minimum USMLE Step 1 Score Requirement: No limits set
Minimum USMLE Step 2 Score Requirement: No limits set
Attempts on any step: No limits set
CS required at time of application: Yes including ECFMG certificate
USCE Requirement: None
Cut-Off time since graduation: No limits set
Program offers couple match: Yes
Visas Sponsored or accepted: No visa

Jackson Memorial Hospital/Jackson Health System Obstetrics and Gynecology Residency Program

Specialty: Obstetrics and Gynecology
Program name: Jackson Memorial Hospital/Jackson Health System Program
Program code: 220-11-21-070
NRMP Code: 1104220C0
Program type: University-based
State: Florida
Address: University of Miami/Jackson Memorial Hospital
          1161 NW 12th Ave, Miami, FL 33136
Phone: (305) 585-5640
Fax: (305) 585-7651
Percentage of IMGs in the program: 30%

Minimum USMLE Step 1 Score Requirement: 220
Minimum USMLE Step 2 Score Requirement: 220
Attempts on any step: Must pass maximum on 2nd attempt including CS exam
CS required at time of application: No
USCE Requirement: None
Cut-Off time since graduation: 10 years
Program offers couple match: Yes
Visas Sponsored or accepted: J1 visa

Georgia

Medical Center of Central Georgia/Mercer University School of Medicine Obstetrics and Gynecology Residency Program

Specialty: Obstetrics and Gynecology
Program name: Medical Center of Central Georgia/Mercer University School of Medicine Program
Program code: 220-12-11-079
State: Georgia
Address: Medical Center of Central Georgia
729 Pine St, Macon, GA 31201

Phone: (478) 633-1056
Percentage of IMGs in the program: 50%
Minimum USMLE Step 1 Score Requirement: No limits set
Minimum USMLE Step 2 Score Requirement: No limits set
Attempts on any step: No limits set
CS required at time of application: Yes
USCE Requirement: None
Cut-Off time since graduation: 10 years
Program offers couple match: Yes
Visas Sponsored or accepted: No visa

Emory University Obstetrics and Gynecology Residency Program

Specialty: Obstetrics and Gynecology
Program name: Emory University Program
Program code: 220-12-21-076
NRMP Code: 1113220C0
Program type: University-based
State: Georgia
Address: Grady Memorial Hospital
          69 Jesse Hill Jr Dr SE, Atlanta, GA 30303
Phone: (404) 251-8800
Fax: (404) 521-3589
Percentage of IMGs in the program: 0% (Occasionally one)

Minimum USMLE Step 1 Score Requirement: 200

Minimum USMLE Step 2 Score Requirement: 210

Attempts on any step: Must pass on first attempt

CS required at time of application: Yes including ECFMG certificate

USCE Requirement: Yes

Cut-Off time since graduation: 5 years

Program offers couple match: Yes

Visas Sponsored or accepted: J1 visa and H1b visa

Medical College of Georgia Obstetrics and Gynecology Residency Program

Specialty: Obstetrics and Gynecology

Program name: Medical College of Georgia Program

Program code: 220-12-21-078

NRMP Code: 1985220C0

State: Georgia

Address: Georgia Regents University MCG
         1120 15th St, Augusta, GA 30912-3305

Phone: (706) 721-2541

Fax: (706) 721-2122

Percentage of IMGs in the program: 10%

Minimum USMLE Step 1 Score Requirement: 200
Minimum USMLE Step 2 Score Requirement: 210
Attempts on any step: Must pass maximum on the 2nd attempt including CS exam
CS required at time of application: Yes including ECFMG certificate
USCE Requirement: Yes
Cut-Off time since graduation: 2 years
Program offers couple match: Yes
Visas Sponsored or accepted: J1 visa

Morehouse School of Medicine Obstetrics and Gynecology Residency Program

Specialty: Obstetrics and Gynecology
Program name: Morehouse School of Medicine Program
Program code: 220-12-21-348
NRMP Code: 2099220C0
Program type: University-based
State: Georgia
Address: Morehouse School of Medicine
720 Westview Dr SW, Atlanta, GA 30310-1495
Phone: (404) 616-1692
Fax: (404) 616-4131

Percentage of IMGs in the program: 0% (Occasionally one)
Minimum USMLE Step 1 Score Requirement: No limits set
Minimum USMLE Step 2 Score Requirement: No limits set
Attempts on any step: No limits set
CS required at time of application: Yes including ECFMG certificate
USCE Requirement: Yes
Cut-Off time since graduation: No limits set
Program offers couple match: No
Visas Sponsored or accepted: J1 visa

Hawaii

University of Hawaii Obstetrics and Gynecology Residency Program

Specialty: Obstetrics and Gynecology
Program name: University of Hawaii Program
Program code: 220-14-31-081
State: Hawaii
Address: Kapiolani Medical Center for Women and Children
  1319 Punahou St, Honolulu, HI 96826
Phone: (808) 203-6518

Fax: (808) 955-2174
Percentage of IMGs in the program: 0%
(Occasionally one)
Minimum USMLE Step 1 Score Requirement:
No limits set
Minimum USMLE Step 2 Score Requirement:
No limits set
Attempts on any step: No limits set
CS required at time of application: Yes
including ECFMG certificate
USCE Requirement: Yes 1year
Cut-Off time since graduation: No limits set
Program offers couple match: Yes
Visas Sponsored or accepted: J1 visa

Illinois

Mount Sinai Hospital Medical Center of Chicago Obstetrics and Gynecology Residency Program

Specialty: Obstetrics and Gynecology
Program name: Mount Sinai Hospital Medical Center of Chicago Program
Program code: 220-16-11-088

NRMP Code: 1144220C0
Program type: Community-based university affiliated hospital
State: Illinois
Address: Mount Sinai Hospital Med Center, Department of Ob/Gyn Rm F208,
           1500 S California Ave, Chicago, IL 60608
Phone: (773) 257-6459
Fax: (773) 257-6359
Percentage of IMGs in the program: 80%
Minimum USMLE Step 1 Score Requirement: No limits set
Minimum USMLE Step 2 Score Requirement: No limits set
Attempts on any step: Must pass on first attempt
CS required at time of application: No
USCE Requirement: None
Cut-Off time since graduation: No limits set
Program offers couple match: Yes
Visas Sponsored or accepted: J1 visa

McGaw Medical Center of Northwestern University Obstetrics and Gynecology Residency Program

Specialty: Obstetrics and Gynecology
Program name: McGaw Medical Center of Northwestern University Program

Program code: 220-16-21-089
NRMP Code: 2247220C0
Program type: University-based
State: Illinois
Address: Prentice Women's Hospital,
        250 E Superior St, Chicago, IL 60611
Phone: (312) 472-4673
Fax: (312) 472-4687
Percentage of IMGs in the program: 5%
Minimum USMLE Step 1 Score Requirement:
No limits set
Minimum USMLE Step 2 Score Requirement:
No limits set
Attempts on any step: Must pass from first
attempt including CS exam
CS required at time of application: No
USCE Requirement: None
Cut-Off time since graduation: No limits set
Program offers couple match: No
Visas Sponsored or accepted: J1 visa and H1b
visa

Rush University Medical Center Obstetrics and Gynecology Residency Program

Specialty: Obstetrics and Gynecology
Program name: Rush University Medical Center
Program
Program code: 220-16-21-090

Program type: University-based
State: Illinois
Address: Rush University Medical Center, 1653 W Congress Pkwy, Chicago, IL 60612-3833
Phone: (312) 942-6610
Fax: (312) 942-6606
Percentage of IMGs in the program: 5%
Minimum USMLE Step 1 Score Requirement: 205
Minimum USMLE Step 2 Score Requirement: 205
Attempts on any step: No limits set
CS required at time of application: No
USCE Requirement: None
Cut-Off time since graduation: 2 years
Program offers couple match: Yes
Visas Sponsored or accepted: J1 visa and H1b visa

Loyola University Obstetrics and Gynecology Residency Program

Specialty: Obstetrics and Gynecology
Program name: Loyola University Program
Program code: 220-16-21-095
NRMP Code: 1170220C0
Program type: University-based
State: Illinois

Address: Loyola University Medical Center,
            2160 S First Ave, Maywood, IL 60153
Phone: (708) 216-8078
Fax: (708) 216-2171
Percentage of IMGs in the program: 5%
Minimum USMLE Step 1 Score Requirement:
No limits set
Minimum USMLE Step 2 Score Requirement:
No limits set
Attempts on any step: Two maximum attempts
including CS exam.
CS required at time of application: No
USCE Requirement: Yes
Cut-Off time since graduation: 5 years
Program offers couple match: Yes
Visas Sponsored or accepted: J1 visa

Southern Illinois University Obstetrics and Gynecology Residency Program

Specialty: Obstetrics and Gynecology
Program name: Southern Illinois University
Program
Program code: 220-16-21-097
NRMP Code: 2922220C0
Program type: Community-based university
affiliated hospital
State: Illinois

Address: Southern Illinois University School of Medicine,

Department of Ob/Gyn PO Box 19640 6W70,

415 N 9th, Springfield, IL 62794-9640

Phone: (217) 545-6498

Fax: (217) 545-7958

Percentage of IMGs in the program: 7%

Minimum USMLE Step 1 Score Requirement: 205

Minimum USMLE Step 2 Score Requirement: 205

Attempts on any step: Must pass on first attempt, might consider 2nd attempt if good score.

CS required at time of application: Yes including ECFMG certificate

USCE Requirement: None

Cut-Off time since graduation: 5 years

Program offers couple match: Yes

Visas Sponsored or accepted: J1 visa

Louisiana

Louisiana State University (Shreveport) Obstetrics and Gynecology Residency Program

Specialty: Obstetrics and Gynecology
Program name: Louisiana State University (Shreveport) Program
Program code: 220-21-11-110
NRMP Code: 1232220C0
Program type: University-based
State: Louisiana
Address: LSU Health Sciences Center Shreveport
    1501 Kings Hwy, Shreveport, LA 71130-3932
Phone: (318) 675-8295
Fax: (318) 675-4671
Percentage of IMGs in the program: 25%
Minimum USMLE Step 1 Score Requirement: No limits set
Minimum USMLE Step 2 Score Requirement: No limits set
Attempts on any step: Must pass on first attempt including CS exam
CS required at time of application: Yes including ECFMG certificate
USCE Requirement: Yes
Cut-Off time since graduation: 5 years
Program offers couple match: Yes
Visas Sponsored or accepted: J1 visa

Louisiana State University (Baton Rouge)Obstetrics and Gynecology Residency Program

Specialty: Obstetrics and Gynecology
Program name: Louisiana State University (Baton Rouge) Program
Program code: 220-21-13-364
NRMP Code: 1221220C0
Program type: University-based
State: Louisiana
Address: Louisiana State University
          500 Rue de la Vie, Baton Rouge, LA 70817
Phone: (225) 215-7442
Fax: (225) 922-3382
Percentage of IMGs in the program: 20%
Minimum USMLE Step 1 Score Requirement: No limits set
Minimum USMLE Step 2 Score Requirement: No limits set
Attempts on any step: No limits set
CS required at time of application: Yes including ECFMG certificate
USCE Requirement: None
Cut-Off time since graduation: No limits set
Program offers couple match: Yes
Visas Sponsored or accepted: J1 visa

Louisiana State University Obstetrics and Gynecology Residency Program

Specialty: Obstetrics and Gynecology
Program name: Louisiana State University Program
Program code: 220-21-21-107
NRMP Code: 1224220C0
Program type: University-based
State: Louisiana
Address: LSU Health Science Center New Orleans
              1542 Tulane Ave, New Orleans, LA 70112
Phone: (504) 568-4890
Fax: (504) 568-6496
Percentage of IMGs in the program: 10%
Minimum USMLE Step 1 Score Requirement: 220
Minimum USMLE Step 2 Score Requirement: 220
Attempts on any step: No limits set
CS required at time of application: Yes including ECFMG certificate
USCE Requirement: Yes 1 month
Cut-Off time since graduation: No limits set
Program offers couple match: Yes
Visas Sponsored or accepted: J1 visa

Ochsner Clinic Foundation Obstetrics and Gynecology Residency Program

Specialty: Obstetrics and Gynecology
Program name: Ochsner Clinic Foundation Program
Program code: 220-21-22-109
NRMP Code: 1966220C0
Program type: Community-based
State: Louisiana
Address: Ochsner Clinic Foundation
2700 Napoleon Ave, New Orleans, LA 70115
Phone: (504) 842-3173
Fax: (504) 842-4152
Percentage of IMGs in the program: 10%
Minimum USMLE Step 1 Score Requirement: No limits set
Minimum USMLE Step 2 Score Requirement: No limits set
Attempts on any step: No limits set
CS required at time of application: Yes including ECFMG certificate
USCE Requirement: None
Cut-Off time since graduation: 5 years
Program offers couple match: Yes
Visas Sponsored or accepted: No visa

Maryland

MedStar Franklin Square Hospital Center Obstetrics and Gynecology Residency Program

Specialty: Obstetrics and Gynecology
Program name: MedStar Franklin Square Hospital Center Program
Program code: 220-23-21-112
NRMP Code: 1240220C0
Program type: Community-based
State: Maryland
Address: MedStar Franklin Square Medical Center
          9000 Franklin Square Dr, Baltimore, MD 21237-3998
Phone: (443) 777-7062
Fax: (443) 777-8180
Percentage of IMGs in the program: 60%
Minimum USMLE Step 1 Score Requirement: No limits set
Minimum USMLE Step 2 Score Requirement: No limits set
Attempts on any step: No limits set
CS required at time of application: No
USCE Requirement: None
Cut-Off time since graduation: No limits set
Program offers couple match: Yes

Visas Sponsored or accepted: J1 visa

Massachusetts

Baystate Medical Center/Tufts University School of Medicine Obstetrics and Gynecology Residency Program

Specialty: Obstetrics and Gynecology
Program name: Baystate Medical Center/Tufts University School of Medicine Program
Program code: 220-24-12-129
NRMP Code: 1286220C0
Program type: Community-based university affiliated hospital
State: Massachusetts
Address: Baystate Medical Center, Department of Ob/Gyn,
759 Chestnut St, Springfield, MA 01199
Phone: (413) 794-5321
Fax: (413) 794-8166
Percentage of IMGs in the program: 20%
Minimum USMLE Step 1 Score Requirement: 220

Minimum USMLE Step 2 Score Requirement:
220
Attempts on any step: Must pass on first
attempt
CS required at time of application: No
USCE Requirement: Yes 1 year
Cut-Off time since graduation: No limits set
Program offers couple match: Yes
Visas Sponsored or accepted: J1 visa

Tufts Medical Center Obstetrics and Gynecology Residency Program

Specialty: Obstetrics and Gynecology
Program name: Tufts Medical Center Program
Program code: 220-24-21-128
NRMP Code: 1263220C0
Program type: University-based
State: Massachusetts
Address: Tufts Medical Center,
          800 Washington St, Boston, MA
02111
Phone: (617) 636-0265
Fax: (617) 636-8315
Percentage of IMGs in the program: 20%
Minimum USMLE Step 1 Score Requirement:
No limits set
Minimum USMLE Step 2 Score Requirement:
No limits set

Attempts on any step: No limits set
CS required at time of application: Yes
including ECFMG certificate
USCE Requirement: None
Cut-Off time since graduation: 6 years
Program offers couple match: Yes
Visas Sponsored or accepted: J1 visa

University of Massachusetts Obstetrics and Gynecology Residency Program

Specialty: Obstetrics and Gynecology
Program name: University of Massachusetts
Program
Program code: 220-24-21-130
NRMP Code: 3050220C0
Program type: University-based
State: Massachusetts
Address: UMass Memorial Medical Center,
Department of Ob/Gyn,
119 Belmont St, Worcester, MA 01605
Phone: (508) 334-8459
Fax: (508) 334-5371
Percentage of IMGs in the program: 10%
Minimum USMLE Step 1 Score Requirement:
No limits set
Minimum USMLE Step 2 Score Requirement:
No limits set

Attempts on any step: Must pass maximum on 2nd attempt
CS required at time of application: Yes including ECFMG certificate
USCE Requirement: Yes, 1 year
Cut-Off time since graduation: No limits set
Program offers couple match: Yes
Visas Sponsored or accepted: J1 visa

Michigan

Henry Ford Hospital/Wayne State University Obstetrics and Gynecology Residency Program

Specialty: Obstetrics and Gynecology
Program name: Henry Ford Hospital/Wayne State University Program
Program code: 220-25-11-136
NRMP Code: 1300220C0
Program type: Community-based university affiliated hospital
State: Michigan
Address: Henry Ford Hospital
          3031 W Grand Blvd, Detroit, MI 48202

Phone: (313) 916-1023
Fax: (313) 916-5008
Percentage of IMGs in the program: 90%
Minimum USMLE Step 1 Score Requirement: 210
Minimum USMLE Step 2 Score Requirement: 210
Attempts on any step: Must pass on the first attempt
CS required at time of application: No but should be scheduled already at time of interview
USCE Requirement: None
Cut-Off time since graduation: 5 years
Program offers couple match: Yes
Visas Sponsored or accepted: J1 visa

St John Hospital and Medical Center Obstetrics and Gynecology Residency Program

Specialty: Obstetrics and Gynecology
Program name: St John Hospital and Medical Center Program
Program code: 220-25-11-137
NRMP Code: 1915220C0
Program type: Community-based university affiliated hospital
State: Michigan

Address: St John Hospital and Medical Center
19251 Mack Ave, Grosse Pointe Woods, MI 48236
Phone: (313) 343-7798
Fax: (313) 343-7840
Percentage of IMGs in the program: 50%
Minimum USMLE Step 1 Score Requirement: No limits set
Minimum USMLE Step 2 Score Requirement: No limits set
Attempts on any step: Must pass on the first attempt
CS required at time of application: No
USCE Requirement: 1 year
Cut-Off time since graduation: 5 years
Program offers couple match: Yes
Visas Sponsored or accepted: J1 visa

William Beaumont Hospital Obstetrics and Gynecology Residency Program

Specialty: Obstetrics and Gynecology
Program name: William Beaumont Hospital Program
Program code: 220-25-11-146
State: Michigan

Address: Beaumont Health System
3535 W 13 Mile Rd, Royal Oak, MI 48073
Phone: (248) 551-0845
Fax: (248) 551-5010
Percentage of IMGs in the program: 15%
Minimum USMLE Step 1 Score Requirement: No limits set
Minimum USMLE Step 2 Score Requirement: No limits set
Attempts on any step: No limits set
CS required at time of application: No
USCE Requirement: None
Cut-Off time since graduation: No limits set
Program offers couple match: Yes
Visas Sponsored or accepted: J1 visa

Grand Rapids Medical Education Partners/Michigan State University Obstetrics and Gynecology Residency Program

Specialty: Obstetrics and Gynecology
Program name: Grand Rapids Medical Education Partners/Michigan State University Program
Program code: 220-25-21-141
NRMP Code: 2077220C0

Program type: Community-based university affiliated hospital
State: Michigan
Address: Grand Rapids Med Education Partners
330 Barclay NE, Grand Rapids, MI 49503
Phone: (616) 391-1929
Fax: (616) 391-3174
Percentage of IMGs in the program: 40%
Minimum USMLE Step 1 Score Requirement: 210
Minimum USMLE Step 2 Score Requirement: 210
Attempts on any step: Must pass on the first attempt
CS required at time of application: No
USCE Requirement: None
Cut-Off time since graduation: 3 years
Program offers couple match: Yes
Visas Sponsored or accepted: J1 visa

Central Michigan University College of Medicine Obstetrics and Gynecology Residency Program

Specialty: Obstetrics and Gynecology
Program name: Central Michigan University College of Medicine Program

Program code: 220-25-21-147
NRMP Code: 1320220C0
Program type: University-based
State: Michigan
Address: Central Michigan University
College of Medicine
            1000 Houghton Ave, Saginaw,
MI 48602
Phone: (989) 583-6828
Fax: (989) 583-6941
Percentage of IMGs in the program: 20%
Minimum USMLE Step 1 Score
Requirement: 210
Minimum USMLE Step 2 Score
Requirement: 210
Attempts on any step: Must pass on the
first attempt
CS required at time of application: Yes
including ECFMG certificate
USCE Requirement: None
Cut-Off time since graduation: 2 years
Program offers couple match: Yes
Visas Sponsored or accepted: J1 visa

Providence Hospital and Medical Centers Obstetrics and Gynecology Residency Program

Specialty: Obstetrics and Gynecology

Program name: Providence Hospital and Medical Centers Program
Program code: 220-25-21-148
NRMP Code: 1303220C0
Program type: Community-based university affiliated hospital
State: Michigan
Address: Providence Hospital and Medical Center
        16001 W Nine Mile Rd, Southfield, MI 48075-4818
Phone: (248) 849-3014
Fax: (248) 849-5398
Percentage of IMGs in the program: 50%
Minimum USMLE Step 1 Score Requirement: 210
Minimum USMLE Step 2 Score Requirement: 210
Attempts on any step: Must pass on the first attempt
CS required at time of application: Yes including ECFMG certificate
USCE Requirement: 1 year
Cut-Off time since graduation: 5 years
Program offers couple match: Yes
Visas Sponsored or accepted: J1 visa

St Joseph Mercy Hospital Obstetrics and Gynecology Residency Program

Specialty: Obstetrics and Gynecology
Program name: St Joseph Mercy Hospital Program
Program code: 220-25-31-131
NRMP Code: 1292220C0
Program type: Community-based university affiliated hospital
State: Michigan
Address: St Joseph Mercy Hospital
      5333 McAuley Dr, Ypsilanti, MI 48197
Phone: (734) 712-5171
Fax: (734) 712-4151
Percentage of IMGs in the program: 20%
Minimum USMLE Step 1 Score Requirement: 210
Minimum USMLE Step 2 Score Requirement: 210
Attempts on any step: No limits set
CS required at time of application: Yes including ECFMG certificate
USCE Requirement: 1-2 months
Cut-Off time since graduation: 2 years
Program offers couple match: Yes
Visas Sponsored or accepted: J1 visa

Oakwood Hospital Obstetrics and Gynecology Residency Program

Specialty: Obstetrics and Gynecology

Program name: Oakwood Hospital Program
Program code: 220-25-31-133
NRMP Code: 1946220C0
Program type: Community-based university affiliated hospital
State: Michigan
Address: Oakwood Hospital and Medical Center
           18101 Oakwood Blvd, Dearborn, MI 48124
Phone: (313) 436-2582
Fax: (313) 436-2783
Percentage of IMGs in the program: 50%
Minimum USMLE Step 1 Score Requirement: 210
Minimum USMLE Step 2 Score Requirement: 210
Attempts on any step: Must pass maximum from the 2nd attempt
CS required at time of application: Yes including ECFMG certificate
USCE Requirement: 1 year
Cut-Off time since graduation: 5 years
Program offers couple match: Yes
Visas Sponsored or accepted: No visa

Hurley Medical Center/Michigan State University Obstetrics and Gynecology Residency Program

Specialty: Obstetrics and Gynecology

Program name: Hurley Medical Center/Michigan State University Program
Program code: 220-25-31-140
NRMP Code: 1307220C0
Program type: Community-based university affiliated hospital
State: Michigan
Address: Hurley Medical Center
One Hurley Plaza, Flint, MI 48503-5993
Phone: (810) 262-6426
Fax: (810) 257-9076
Percentage of IMGs in the program: 80%
Minimum USMLE Step 1 Score Requirement: 215
Minimum USMLE Step 2 Score Requirement: 220
Attempts on any step: Must pass maximum from the 2nd attempt
CS required at time of application: Yes including ECFMG certificate
USCE Requirement: None
Cut-Off time since graduation: 7 years
Program offers couple match: Yes
Visas Sponsored or accepted: J1 visa

Sparrow Hospital/Michigan State University Obstetrics and Gynecology Residency Program

Specialty: Obstetrics and Gynecology
Program name: Sparrow Hospital/Michigan State University Program
Program code: 220-25-31-143
NRMP Code: 1315220C0
Program type: Community-based university affiliated hospital
State: Michigan
Address: Sparrow Hospital
        1215 E Michigan Ave, Lansing, MI 48909-7980
Phone: (517) 364-2577
Fax: (517) 364-2222
Percentage of IMGs in the program: 40%
Minimum USMLE Step 1 Score Requirement: 210
Minimum USMLE Step 2 Score Requirement: 210
Attempts on any step: No limits set
CS required at time of application: Yes including ECFMG certificate
USCE Requirement: None unless you graduated more than 2 years ago
Cut-Off time since graduation: None but must be clinically active within the last 2 years
Program offers couple match: Yes
Visas Sponsored or accepted: J1 visa

Detroit Medical Center/Wayne State University Obstetrics and Gynecology Residency Program

Specialty: Obstetrics and Gynecology
Program name: Detroit Medical Center/Wayne State University Program
Program code: 220-25-31-358
NRMP Code: 1295220C0
Program type: University-based
State: Michigan
Address: Hutzel Women's Hospital
　　　　　3990 John R St, Detroit, MI 48021
Phone: (313) 993-4030
Fax: (313) 993-4116
Percentage of IMGs in the program: 30%
Minimum USMLE Step 1 Score Requirement: No limits set
Minimum USMLE Step 2 Score Requirement: No limits set
Attempts on any step: Must pass on the first attempt
CS required at time of application: Yes including ECFMG certificate
USCE Requirement: None
Cut-Off time since graduation: 5 years
Program offers couple match: Yes
Visas Sponsored or accepted: J1 visa

Minnesota

Mayo Clinic College of Medicine (Rochester) Obstetrics and Gynecology Residency Program

Specialty: Obstetrics and Gynecology
Program name: Mayo Clinic College of Medicine (Rochester) Program
Program code: 220-26-21-150
NRMP Code: 1328220C1, 1328220C0
Program type: University-based
State: Minnesota
Address: Mayo Clinic
200 First St SW, Rochester, MN 55905
Phone: (507) 266-3262
Fax: (507) 266-7953
Percentage of IMGs in the program: 20%
Minimum USMLE Step 1 Score Requirement: 215
Minimum USMLE Step 2 Score Requirement: 215
Attempts on any step: Must pass on the first attempt
CS required at time of application: Yes including ECFMG certificate

USCE Requirement: 2 months
Cut-Off time since graduation: 10 years
Program offers couple match: Yes
Visas Sponsored or accepted: J1 visa and H1b visa

Mississippi

University of Mississippi Medical Center Obstetrics and Gynecology Residency Program

Specialty: Obstetrics and Gynecology
Program name: University of Mississippi Medical Center Program
Program code: 220-27-11-151
NRMP Code: 1957220C0
Program type: University-based
State: Mississippi
Address: University of Mississippi Medical Center
         2500 N State St, Jackson, MS 39216
Phone: (601) 984-5339
Fax: (601) 984-4566
Percentage of IMGs in the program: 10%

Minimum USMLE Step 1 Score Requirement:
220
Minimum USMLE Step 2 Score Requirement:
220
Attempts on any step: No limits set
CS required at time of application: No
USCE Requirement: None
Cut-Off time since graduation: No limits set
Program offers couple match: Yes
Visas Sponsored or accepted: J1 visa

Missouri

University of Missouri at Kansas City Obstetrics and Gynecology Residency Program

Specialty: Obstetrics and Gynecology
Program name: University of Missouri at Kansas City Program
Program code: 220-28-21-154
NRMP Code: 1343220C0,
Program type: Community-based university affiliated hospital
State: Missouri

Address: Truman Medical Center
2301 Holmes St, Kansas City, MO 64108
Phone: (816) 404-0886
Fax: (816) 404-0888
Percentage of IMGs in the program: 10%
Minimum USMLE Step 1 Score Requirement: No limits set
Minimum USMLE Step 2 Score Requirement: No limits set
Attempts on any step: No limits set
CS required at time of application: Yes including ECFMG certificate
USCE Requirement: None
Cut-Off time since graduation: 3 years
Program offers couple match: Yes
Visas Sponsored or accepted: J1 visa

Mercy Hospital (St Louis) Obstetrics and Gynecology Residency Program

Specialty: Obstetrics and Gynecology
Program name: Mercy Hospital (St Louis) Program
Program code: 220-28-22-157
NRMP Code: 1362220C0
Program type: Community-based
State: Missouri

Address: Mercy Hospital St Louis
615 S New Ballas Rd, St Louis, MO 63141
Phone: (314) 251-6826
Fax: (314) 251-4376
Percentage of IMGs in the program: 5%
Minimum USMLE Step 1 Score Requirement: 220
Minimum USMLE Step 2 Score Requirement: 220
Attempts on any step: Must pass on the first attempt
CS required at time of application: No
USCE Requirement: None
Cut-Off time since graduation: 5 years
Program offers couple match: Yes
Visas Sponsored or accepted: H1b visa

Nebraska

Creighton University Obstetrics and Gynecology Residency Program

Specialty: Obstetrics and Gynecology OB GYN Residency
Program name: Creighton University Program
Program code: 220-30-21-160

NRMP Code: 1372220C0
Program type: University-based
State: Nebraska
Address: Alegent Creighton University Medical Center

       601 N 30th St, Omaha, NE 68131
Phone: (402) 280-4438
Fax: (402) 280-4315
Percentage of IMGs in the program: 5%
Minimum USMLE Step 1 Score Requirement: No limits set
Minimum USMLE Step 2 Score Requirement: No limits set
Attempts on any step: No limits set
CS required at time of application: No
USCE Requirement: None
Cut-Off time since graduation: No limits set
Program offers couple match: Yes
Visas Sponsored or accepted: No visa

Nevada

University of Nevada School of Medicine (Las Vegas) Obstetrics and Gynecology Residency Program

Specialty: Obstetrics and Gynecology OB GYN Residency
Program name: University of Nevada School of Medicine (Las Vegas) Program
Program code: 220-31-21-318
NRMP Code: 2028220C0
Program type: Community-based university affiliated hospital
State: Nevada
Address: University of Nevada School of Medicine
2040 W Charleston Blvd, Las Vegas, NV 89102
Phone: (702) 671-2385
Fax: (702) 671-2333
Percentage of IMGs in the program: 20%
Minimum USMLE Step 1 Score Requirement: No limits set
Minimum USMLE Step 2 Score Requirement: No limits set
Attempts on any step: No limits set
CS required at time of application: Yes including ECFMG certificate
USCE Requirement: None
Cut-Off time since graduation: 5 years
Program offers couple match: Yes
Visas Sponsored or accepted: J1 visa

New Hampshire

Dartmouth-Hitchcock Medical Center Obstetrics and Gynecology Residency Program

Specialty: Obstetrics and Gynecology OB GYN Residency
Program name: Dartmouth-Hitchcock Medical Center Program
Program code: 220-32-12-352
NRMP Code: 1377220C0
Program type: University-based
State: New Hampshire
Address: Dartmouth-Hitchcock Medical Center One Medical Center Dr, Lebanon, NH 03756
Phone: (603) 653-9289
Fax: (603) 650-0906
Percentage of IMGs in the program: 0% (occasionally 1 match)
Minimum USMLE Step 1 Score Requirement: No limits set
Minimum USMLE Step 2 Score Requirement: No limits set
Attempts on any step: Must pass on the first attempt

CS required at time of application: Yes including ECFMG certificate
USCE Requirement: 2-3 months (Canadian or European rotations are accepted)
Cut-Off time since graduation: 3 years
Program offers couple match: Yes
Visas Sponsored or accepted: J1 visa

New Jersey

Cooper Medical School of Rowan University/Cooper University Hospital Obstetrics and Gynecology Residency Program

Specialty: Obstetrics and Gynecology OB GYN Residency
Program name: Cooper Medical School of Rowan University/Cooper University Hospital Program
Program code: 220-33-11-162
NRMP Code: 1380220C0
Program type: University-based
State: New Jersey
Address: Cooper Hospital-University Medical Centre
            3 Cooper Plaza, Camden, NJ 08103

Phone: (856) 342-2965
Fax: (856) 365-1967
Percentage of IMGs in the program: 25%
Minimum USMLE Step 1 Score Requirement:
No limits set
Minimum USMLE Step 2 Score Requirement:
No limits set
Attempts on any step: No limits set
CS required at time of application: Yes
including ECFMG certificate
USCE Requirement: None
Cut-Off time since graduation: 5 years
Program offers couple match: Yes
Visas Sponsored or accepted: J1 visa

Monmouth Medical Center Obstetrics and Gynecology Residency Program

Specialty: Obstetrics and Gynecology OB GYN
Residency
Program name: Monmouth Medical Center
Program
Program code: 220-33-11-164
State: New Jersey
Address: Monmouth Medical Center
300 Second Ave, Long Branch, NJ
07740
Phone: (732) 923-6795
Fax: (732) 923-6793

Percentage of IMGs in the program: 80%
Minimum USMLE Step 1 Score Requirement:
No limits set
Minimum USMLE Step 2 Score Requirement:
No limits set
Attempts on any step: Must pass maximum on
the 3rd attempt
CS required at time of application: No
USCE Requirement: None
Cut-Off time since graduation: No limits set
Program offers couple match: No
Visas Sponsored or accepted: No visa

St Barnabas Medical Center Obstetrics and Gynecology Residency Program

Specialty: Obstetrics and Gynecology OB GYN
Residency
Program name: St Barnabas Medical Center
Program
Program code: 220-33-12-163
NRMP Code: 1396220C0
Program type: Community-based university
affiliated hospital
State: New Jersey
Address: St Barnabas Medical Center
          94 Old Short Hills Rd, Livingston, NJ
07039
Phone: (973) 322-5281

Fax: (973) 533-4492
Percentage of IMGs in the program: 50%
Minimum USMLE Step 1 Score Requirement:
No limits set
Minimum USMLE Step 2 Score Requirement:
No limits set
Attempts on any step: No limits set
CS required at time of application: No
USCE Requirement: Yes
Cut-Off time since graduation: No limits set
Program offers couple match: Yes
Visas Sponsored or accepted: J1 visa

Jersey Shore University Medical Center Obstetrics and Gynecology Residency Program

Specialty: Obstetrics and Gynecology OB GYN
Residency
Program name: Jersey Shore University Medical
Center Program
Program code: 220-33-12-165
NRMP Code: 1395220C0
Program type: Community-based university
affiliated hospital
State: New Jersey
Address: Jersey Shore University Medical
Center
        1945 State Rte 33, Neptune, NJ 07754
Phone: (732) 776-3790

Fax: (732) 776-4525
Percentage of IMGs in the program: 40%
Minimum USMLE Step 1 Score Requirement: No limits set
Minimum USMLE Step 2 Score Requirement: No limits set
Attempts on any step: Must pass on the first attempt
CS required at time of application: Yes including ECFMG certificate
USCE Requirement: None
Cut-Off time since graduation: No limits set
Program offers couple match: Yes
Visas Sponsored or accepted: No visa

Saint Peter's University Hospital/Rutgers Robert Wood Johnson Medical School Obstetrics and Gynecology Residency Program

Specialty: Obstetrics and Gynecology OB GYN Residency
Program name: Saint Peter's University Hospital/Rutgers Robert Wood Johnson Medical School Program
Program code: 220-33-12-362
NRMP Code: 3211220C0
Program type: Community-based university affiliated hospital

State: New Jersey
Address: St Peter's University Hospital
254 Easton Ave, New Brunswick, NJ 08901
Phone: (732) 565-5415
Fax: (732) 342-8479
Percentage of IMGs in the program: 60%
Minimum USMLE Step 1 Score Requirement: No limits set
Minimum USMLE Step 2 Score Requirement: No limits set
Attempts on any step: No limits set
CS required at time of application: Yes including ECFMG certificate
USCE Requirement: None
Cut-Off time since graduation: No limits set
Program offers couple match: Yes
Visas Sponsored or accepted: J1 visa

Rutgers Robert Wood Johnson Medical School Obstetrics and Gynecology Residency Program

Specialty: Obstetrics and Gynecology OB GYN Residency
Program name: Rutgers Robert Wood Johnson Medical School Program
Program code: 220-33-21-167

NRMP Code: 2918220C0
Program type: University-based
State: New Jersey
Address: Rutgers Robert Wood Johnson
Medical School
          125 Paterson St, New Brunswick, NJ
08901
Phone: (732) 235-6375
Fax: (732) 235-9855
Percentage of IMGs in the program: 15%
Minimum USMLE Step 1 Score Requirement:
No limits set
Minimum USMLE Step 2 Score Requirement:
No limits set
Attempts on any step: No limits set
CS required at time of application: Yes
including ECFMG certificate
USCE Requirement: None
Cut-Off time since graduation: No limits set
Program offers couple match: Yes
Visas Sponsored or accepted: J1 visa

Newark Beth Israel Medical Center Obstetrics and Gynecology Residency Program

Specialty: Obstetrics and Gynecology OB
GYN Residency
Program name: Newark Beth Israel
Medical Center Program

Program code: 220-33-21-321
NRMP Code: 1397220P0, 1397220C0
Program type: Community-based
State: New Jersey
Address: Newark Beth Israel Medical Center
201 Lyons Ave, Newark, NJ 07112-2027
Phone: (973) 926-4882
Fax: (973) 923-7497
Percentage of IMGs in the program: 50%
Minimum USMLE Step 1 Score Requirement: No limits set
Minimum USMLE Step 2 Score Requirement: No limits set
Attempts on any step: Must pass on the first attempt
CS required at time of application: Yes including ECFMG certificate
USCE Requirement: Yes
Cut-Off time since graduation: 5 years
Program offers couple match: No
Visas Sponsored or accepted: No visa

New York Medical College at St Joseph's Regional Medical Center Obstetrics and Gynecology Residency Program

Specialty: Obstetrics and Gynecology OB GYN Residency
Program name: New York Medical College at St Joseph's Regional Medical Center Program
Program code: 220-33-21-323
NRMP Code: 1406220C0
Program type: Community-based university affiliated hospital
State: New Jersey
Address: St Joseph's Regional Medical Center
703 Main St, Paterson, NJ 07503
Phone: (973) 754-2726
Fax: (973) 754-2725
Percentage of IMGs in the program: 90%
Minimum USMLE Step 1 Score Requirement: No limits set
Minimum USMLE Step 2 Score Requirement: No limits set
Attempts on any step: Must pass on the first attempt
CS required at time of application: Yes including ECFMG certificate
USCE Requirement: None
Cut-Off time since graduation: 5 years
Program offers couple match: Yes
Visas Sponsored or accepted: J1 visa

Newark Beth Israel Medical Center (Jersey City) Obstetrics and Gynecology Residency Program

Specialty: Obstetrics and Gynecology OB GYN Residency
Program name: Newark Beth Israel Medical Center (Jersey City) Program
Program code: 220-33-21-324
NRMP Code: 1390220C0
Program type: Community-based
State: New Jersey
Address: Jersey City Medical Center
         355 Grand St, Jersey City, NJ 07302
Phone: (201) 915-2462
Fax: (201) 915-2481
Percentage of IMGs in the program: 60%
Minimum USMLE Step 1 Score Requirement: No limits set
Minimum USMLE Step 2 Score Requirement: No limits set
Attempts on any step: Must pass maximum on the 2nd attempt
CS required at time of application: Yes including ECFMG certificate
USCE Requirement: None
Cut-Off time since graduation: 7 years
Program offers couple match: Yes
Visas Sponsored or accepted: J1 visa

Rutgers New Jersey Medical School Obstetrics and Gynecology Residency Program

Specialty: Obstetrics and Gynecology OB GYN Residency
Program name: Rutgers New Jersey Medical School Program
Program code: 220-33-31-166
NRMP Code: 1398220C0,
Program type: University-based
State: New Jersey
Address: Rutgers New Jersey Medical School
            185 S Orange Ave, Newark, NJ 07103-2714
Phone: (973) 972-5266
Fax: (973) 972-4574
Percentage of IMGs in the program: 30%
Minimum USMLE Step 1 Score Requirement: No limits set
Minimum USMLE Step 2 Score Requirement: No limits set
Attempts on any step: No limits set
CS required at time of application: Yes including ECFMG certificate
USCE Requirement: None
Cut-Off time since graduation: No limits set
Program offers couple match: No
Visas Sponsored or accepted: J1 visa

Atlantic Health (Morristown) Obstetrics and Gynecology Residency Program

Specialty: Obstetrics and Gynecology OB GYN Residency
Program name: Atlantic Health (Morristown) Program
Program code: 220-33-31-365
NRMP Code:
Program type:
State: New Jersey
Address: Morristown Medical Center
100 Madison Ave, Morristown, NJ 07962-1956
Phone: (973) 971-6279
Fax: (973) 290-7054
Percentage of IMGs in the program: 50%
Minimum USMLE Step 1 Score Requirement: 220
Minimum USMLE Step 2 Score Requirement: 220
Attempts on any step: Must pass on the first attempt
CS required at time of application: Yes including ECFMG certificate
USCE Requirement: None
Cut-Off time since graduation: 5 years
Program offers couple match: No
Visas Sponsored or accepted: J1 visa

New Mexico

University of New Mexico Obstetrics and Gynecology Residency Program

Specialty: Obstetrics and Gynecology OB GYN Residency
Program name: University of New Mexico Program
Program code: 220-34-21-169
NRMP Code: 1962220C0
Program type: University-based
State: New Mexico
Address: University of New Mexico Health Science Center
            1 University of New Mexico, Albuquerque, NM 87131-0001
Phone: (505) 272-6883
Fax: (505) 272-3918
Percentage of IMGs in the program: 5%
Minimum USMLE Step 1 Score Requirement: 225
Minimum USMLE Step 2 Score Requirement: 225
Attempts on any step: No limits set

CS required at time of application: Yes
including ECFMG certificate
USCE Requirement: None
Cut-Off time since graduation: No limits set
Program offers couple match: Yes
Visas Sponsored or accepted: J1 visa

New York

Icahn School of Medicine at Mount Sinai (Beth Israel) Obstetrics and Gynecology Residency Program

Specialty: Obstetrics and Gynecology
Program name: Icahn School of Medicine at Mount Sinai (Beth Israel) Program
Program code: 220-35-11-179
NRMP Code: 1470220C0
Program type: Community-based university affiliated hospital
State: New York
Address: Beth Israel Medical Center
350 E 17th St, New York, NY 10003
Phone: (212) 420-4548

Fax: (212) 420-2980
Percentage of IMGs in the program: 10%
Minimum USMLE Step 1 Score Requirement: 220
Minimum USMLE Step 2 Score Requirement: 220
Attempts on any step: Must pass on first attempt
CS required at time of application: Yes including ECFMG certificate
USCE Requirement: Yes however 1-2 years OBGYN experience outside the states is also considered
Cut-Off time since graduation: No limits set
Program offers couple match: Yes
Visas Sponsored or accepted: J1 visa and H1b visa

Bronx-Lebanon Hospital Center Obstetrics and Gynecology Residency Program

Specialty: Obstetrics and Gynecology
Program name: Bronx-Lebanon Hospital Center Program
Program code: 220-35-11-180
State: New York
Address: Bronx-Lebanon Hospital Center
        1650 Grand Concourse Ave, Bronx, NY 10457

Phone: (718) 239-8384
Fax: (718) 239-8360
Percentage of IMGs in the program: 70%
Minimum USMLE Step 1 Score Requirement: 205
Minimum USMLE Step 2 Score Requirement: 205
Attempts on any step: No limits set
CS required at time of application: Yes including ECFMG certificate
USCE Requirement: None
Cut-Off time since graduation: No limits set
Program offers couple match: Yes
Visas Sponsored or accepted: J1 visa and H1b visa

Flushing Hospital Medical Center Obstetrics and Gynecology Residency Program

Specialty: Obstetrics and Gynecology
Program name: Flushing Hospital Medical Center Program
Program code: 220-35-11-184
NRMP Code: 1445220P0, 1445220C0
Program type: Community-based
State: New York
Address: Flushing Hospital Medical Center
4500 Parsons Blvd, Flushing, NY 11355

Phone: (718) 670-5440
Fax: (718) 670-5780
Percentage of IMGs in the program: 100%
Minimum USMLE Step 1 Score Requirement:
No limits set
Minimum USMLE Step 2 Score Requirement:
No limits set
Attempts on any step: No limits set
CS required at time of application: Yes
including ECFMG certificate
USCE Requirement: None
Cut-Off time since graduation: No limits set
Program offers couple match: No
Visas Sponsored or accepted: J1 visa

NSLIJ/Hofstra North Shore-LIJ School of Medicine at Lenox Hill Hospital Obstetrics and Gynecology Residency Program

Specialty: Obstetrics and Gynecology
Program name: NSLIJ/Hofstra North Shore-LIJ
School of Medicine at Lenox Hill Hospital
Program
Program code: 220-35-11-188
NRMP Code: 1483220C0
Program type: Community-based University
affiliated hospital
State: New York

Address: Lenox Hill Hospital
130 E 77th St, New York, NY 10021-1883
Phone: (212) 434-2160
Fax: (212) 434-2180
Percentage of IMGs in the program: 20%
Minimum USMLE Step 1 Score Requirement: No limits set
Minimum USMLE Step 2 Score Requirement: No limits set
Attempts on any step: No limits set
CS required at time of application: No
USCE Requirement: None
Cut-Off time since graduation: No limits set
Program offers couple match: Yes
Visas Sponsored or accepted: J1 visa and H1b visa

Lutheran Medical Center Obstetrics and Gynecology Residency Program

Specialty: Obstetrics and Gynecology
Program name: Lutheran Medical Center Program
Program code: 220-35-11-191
NRMP Code: 1430220C0
Program type: Community-based University affiliated hospital
State: New York

Address: Lutheran Medical Center
        150 55th St, Brooklyn, NY 11220
Phone: (718) 630-6834
Fax: (718) 630-7865
Percentage of IMGs in the program: 15%
Minimum USMLE Step 1 Score Requirement: 210
Minimum USMLE Step 2 Score Requirement: 210
Attempts on any step: No limits set
CS required at time of application: Yes including ECFMG certificate
USCE Requirement: None
Cut-Off time since graduation: No limits set
Program offers couple match: Yes
Visas Sponsored or accepted: J1 visa and H1b visa

Icahn School of Medicine at Mount Sinai/St Luke's-Roosevelt Hospital Center Obstetrics and Gynecology Residency Program

Specialty: Obstetrics and Gynecology
Program name: Icahn School of Medicine at Mount Sinai/St Luke's-Roosevelt Hospital Center Program
Program code: 220-35-11-204
NRMP Code: 2070220C0
Program type: Community-based university

affiliated hospital
State: New York
Address: St Lukes-Roosevelt Hospital Center
            1000 Tenth Ave, New York, NY 10019
Phone: (212) 523-8366
Fax: (212) 523-8066
Percentage of IMGs in the program: 10%
(variable)
Minimum USMLE Step 1 Score Requirement:
230
Minimum USMLE Step 2 Score Requirement:
220
Attempts on any step: Must pass maximum on
the 2nd attempt
CS required at time of application: Yes
including ECFMG certificate
USCE Requirement: None
Cut-Off time since graduation: No limits set
Program offers couple match: Yes
Visas Sponsored or accepted: J1 visa and H1b
visa

Staten Island University Hospital Obstetrics and Gynecology Residency Program

Specialty: Obstetrics and Gynecology
Program name: Staten Island University
Hospital Program
Program code: 220-35-11-207

NRMP Code: 1515220C0
Program type: Community-based University affiliated hospital
State: New York
Address: Staten Island University Hospital
       475 Seaview Ave, Staten Island, NY 10305
Phone: (718) 226-8074
Fax: (718) 226-6873
Percentage of IMGs in the program: 60%
Minimum USMLE Step 1 Score Requirement: No limits set
Minimum USMLE Step 2 Score Requirement: No limits set
Attempts on any step: No limits set
CS required at time of application: Yes including ECFMG certificate
USCE Requirement: None
Cut-Off time since graduation: No limits set
Program offers couple match: Yes
Visas Sponsored or accepted: J1 visa and H1b visa

Brooklyn Hospital Center Obstetrics and Gynecology Residency Program

Specialty: Obstetrics and Gynecology
Program name: Brooklyn Hospital Center Program

Program code: 220-35-12-182
NRMP Code: 1420220C0
Program type: Community-based university affiliated hospital
State: New York
Address: Brooklyn Hospital Center
   121 DeKalb Ave, Brooklyn, NY 11201
Phone: (718) 250-8322
Fax: (718) 250-8881
Percentage of IMGs in the program: 100%
Minimum USMLE Step 1 Score Requirement: No limits set
Minimum USMLE Step 2 Score Requirement: No limits set
Attempts on any step: No limits set
CS required at time of application: Yes including ECFMG certificate
USCE Requirement: None
Cut-Off time since graduation: No limits set
Program offers couple match: Yes
Visas Sponsored or accepted: J1 visa and H1b visa

Richmond University Medical Center Obstetrics and Gynecology Residency Program

Specialty: Obstetrics and Gynecology
Program name: Richmond University Medical Center Program

Program code: 220-35-12-206
State: New York
Address: Richmond University Medical Center
        355 Bard Ave, Staten Island, NY 10310
Phone: (718) 818-4273
Fax: (718) 818-3943
Percentage of IMGs in the program: 50%
Minimum USMLE Step 1 Score Requirement:
No limits set
Minimum USMLE Step 2 Score Requirement:
No limits set
Attempts on any step: No limits set
CS required at time of application: Yes
including ECFMG certificate
USCE Requirement: None
Cut-Off time since graduation: No limits set
Program offers couple match: Yes
Visas Sponsored or accepted: J1 visa and H1b
visa

University at Buffalo (Sisters of Charity) Obstetrics and Gynecology Residency Program

Specialty: Obstetrics and Gynecology
Program name: University at Buffalo (Sisters of
Charity) Program
Program code: 220-35-21-171
State: New York

Address: Sisters of Charity Hospital
          2157 Main St, Buffalo, NY 14214
Phone: (716) 862-1589
Fax: (716) 862-1881
Percentage of IMGs in the program: 20%
Minimum USMLE Step 1 Score Requirement:
No limits set
Minimum USMLE Step 2 Score Requirement:
No limits set
Attempts on any step: No limits set
CS required at time of application: No
USCE Requirement: None
Cut-Off time since graduation: No limits set
Program offers couple match: Yes
Visas Sponsored or accepted: No visa

University at Buffalo Obstetrics and Gynecology Residency Program

Specialty: Obstetrics and Gynecology
Program name: University at Buffalo Program
Program code: 220-35-21-172
NRMP Code: 3099220C0
Program type: University-based
State: New York
Address: Women and Children's Hospital of Buffalo
          219 Bryant St, Buffalo, NY 14222
Phone: (716) 878-7750

Fax: (716) 888-3833
Percentage of IMGs in the program: 50%
Minimum USMLE Step 1 Score Requirement: No limits set
Minimum USMLE Step 2 Score Requirement: No limits set
Attempts on any step: No limits set
CS required at time of application: No
USCE Requirement: None
Cut-Off time since graduation: No limits set
Program offers couple match: Yes
Visas Sponsored or accepted: J1 visa

Albert Einstein College of Medicine Obstetrics and Gynecology Residency Program

Specialty: Obstetrics and Gynecology
Program name: Albert Einstein College of Medicine Program
Program code: 220-35-21-178
NRMP Code: 3153220C0
Program type: University-based
State: New York
Address: Albert Einstein College of Medicine
              1300 Morris Park Ave, Bronx, NY 10461
Phone: (718) 430-4031
Fax: (718) 430-8774
Percentage of IMGs in the program: 20%

Minimum USMLE Step 1 Score Requirement:
No limits set
Minimum USMLE Step 2 Score Requirement:
No limits set
Attempts on any step: Preferably no failures
CS required at time of application: No
USCE Requirement: None
Cut-Off time since graduation: No limits set
Program offers couple match: Yes
Visas Sponsored or accepted: J1 visa and H1b

Jamaica Hospital Medical Center Obstetrics and Gynecology Residency Program

Specialty: Obstetrics and Gynecology
Program name: Jamaica Hospital Medical Center Program
Program code: 220-35-21-186
NRMP Code: 1449220C0, 1449220P0
Program type: Community-based
State: New York
Address: Jamaica Hospital Medical Center
8900 Van Wyck Expwy, Jamaica, NY 11418
Phone: (718) 206-6808
Fax: (718) 206-6829
Percentage of IMGs in the program: 100%

Minimum USMLE Step 1 Score Requirement:
No limits set
Minimum USMLE Step 2 Score Requirement:
No limits set
Attempts on any step: Prefer passage on first attempt but not strict
CS required at time of application: Yes including ECFMG certificate
USCE Requirement: Yes at least 1-2 months within the last 2 years
Cut-Off time since graduation: 5 years
Program offers couple match: Yes
Visas Sponsored or accepted: J1 visa

Icahn School of Medicine at Mount Sinai Obstetrics and Gynecology Residency Program

Specialty: Obstetrics and Gynecology
Program name: Icahn School of Medicine at Mount Sinai Program
Program code: 220-35-21-196
NRMP Code: 1490220C0, 1490220P0
Program type: University-based
State: New York
Address: Mount Sinai Medical Center
         One Gustave L Levy Pl, New York, NY 10029
Phone: (212) 241-8578

Fax: (212) 241-3833
Percentage of IMGs in the program: 15% (Variable)
Minimum USMLE Step 1 Score Requirement: 200
Minimum USMLE Step 2 Score Requirement: 205
Attempts on any step: Must pass on first attempt
CS required at time of application: Yes including ECFMG certificate
USCE Requirement: Yes but 1-2 years experience outside the US is considered
Cut-Off time since graduation: No limits set
Program offers couple match: Yes
Visas Sponsored or accepted: J1 visa and H1b visa

New York Presbyterian Hospital (Cornell Campus) Obstetrics and Gynecology Residency Program

Specialty: Obstetrics and Gynecology
Program name: New York Presbyterian Hospital (Cornell Campus) Program
Program code: 220-35-21-197
NRMP Code: 1492220C0, 1492220P0
Program type: University-based
State: New York

Address: New York Presbyterian Hospital-Cornell

       525 E 68th St, New York, NY 10065

Phone: (212) 746-3058

Fax: (212) 746-8490

Percentage of IMGs in the program: 5% (Variable)

Minimum USMLE Step 1 Score Requirement: No limits set

Minimum USMLE Step 2 Score Requirement: No limits set

Attempts on any step: No limits set

CS required at time of application: Yes including ECFMG certificate

USCE Requirement: None

Cut-Off time since graduation: No limits set

Program offers couple match: Yes

Visas Sponsored or accepted: J1 visa

New York Medical College at Westchester Medical Center Obstetrics and Gynecology Residency Program

Specialty: Obstetrics and Gynecology

Program name: New York Medical College at Westchester Medical Center Program

Program code: 220-35-21-199

NRMP Code: 1443220P0, 1443220C0

Program type: University-based
State: New York
Address: Metropolitan Hospital Center
           1901 First Ave, New York, NY 10029
Phone: (212) 423-6796   Ext: 6796
Fax: (212) 423-8121
Percentage of IMGs in the program: 0%
(Occasionally one)
Minimum USMLE Step 1 Score Requirement:
No limits set
Minimum USMLE Step 2 Score Requirement:
No limits set
Attempts on any step: No limits set
CS required at time of application: Yes
including ECFMG certificate
USCE Requirement: None
Cut-Off time since graduation: No limits set
Program offers couple match: Yes
Visas Sponsored or accepted: No visa

New York University School of Medicine Obstetrics and Gynecology Residency Program

Specialty: Obstetrics and Gynecology
Program name: New York University School of
Medicine Program
Program code: 220-35-21-200
NRMP Code: 2978220C0

Program type: University-based
State: New York
Address: New York University Medical Center
          550 First Ave, New York, NY 10016
Phone: (212) 263-6453
Fax: (212) 263-8251
Percentage of IMGs in the program: 8%
Minimum USMLE Step 1 Score Requirement:
No limits set
Minimum USMLE Step 2 Score Requirement:
No limits set
Attempts on any step: No limits set
CS required at time of application: Yes
including ECFMG certificate
USCE Requirement: None
Cut-Off time since graduation: No limits set
Program offers couple match: Yes
Visas Sponsored or accepted: J1 visa and H1b
visa

SUNY Health Science Center at Brooklyn Obstetrics and Gynecology Residency Program

Specialty: Obstetrics and Gynecology
Program name: SUNY Health Science Center at
Brooklyn Program
Program code: 220-35-21-208
State: New York

Address: SUNY Downstate Medical Center
450 Clarkson Ave, Brooklyn, NY 11203-2098
Phone: (718) 270-3320
Fax: (718) 270-4122
Percentage of IMGs in the program: 40%
Minimum USMLE Step 1 Score Requirement: No limits set
Minimum USMLE Step 2 Score Requirement: No limits set
Attempts on any step: No limits set
CS required at time of application: No
USCE Requirement: None
Cut-Off time since graduation: No limits set
Program offers couple match: Yes
Visas Sponsored or accepted: J1 visa and H1b visa

University of Rochester Obstetrics and Gynecology Residency Program

Specialty: Obstetrics and Gynecology
Program name: University of Rochester Program
Program code: 220-35-21-213
NRMP Code: 1511220C0
Program type: University-based
State: New York

Address: University of Rochester Medical Center
         601 Elmwood Ave Rochester, NY 14642-8668
Phone: (585) 275-3733
Fax: (585) 756-4967
Percentage of IMGs in the program: 0% (Occasionally one)
Minimum USMLE Step 1 Score Requirement: No limits set
Minimum USMLE Step 2 Score Requirement: No limits set
Attempts on any step: No limits set
CS required at time of application: Yes including ECFMG certificate
USCE Requirement: None
Cut-Off time since graduation: 5 years
Program offers couple match: Yes
Visas Sponsored or accepted: J1 visa

SUNY Upstate Medical University Obstetrics and Gynecology Residency Program

Specialty: Obstetrics and Gynecology
Program name: SUNY Upstate Medical University Program
Program code: 220-35-21-215
NRMP Code: 1516220C0

Program type: University-based
State: New York
Address: SUNY Upstate Medical Center
750 E Adams St, Syracuse, NY 13210
Phone: (315) 464-5692
Percentage of IMGs in the program: 0%-40%
(Varies from year to year)
Minimum USMLE Step 1 Score Requirement:
No limits set
Minimum USMLE Step 2 Score Requirement:
No limits set
Attempts on any step: No limits set
CS required at time of application: Yes
including ECFMG certificate
USCE Requirement: None
Cut-Off time since graduation: No limits set but
recent clinical experience required
Program offers couple match: Yes
Visas Sponsored or accepted: J1 visa

Lincoln Medical and Mental Health Center Obstetrics and Gynecology Residency Program

Specialty: Obstetrics and Gynecology
Program name: Lincoln Medical and Mental
Health Center Program
Program code: 220-35-21-326
State: New York

Address: Lincoln Medical and Mental Health Center

        234 E 149th St, Bronx, NY 10451

Phone: (718) 579-5830

Fax: (718) 579-4699

Percentage of IMGs in the program: 40%

Minimum USMLE Step 1 Score Requirement: 205

Minimum USMLE Step 2 Score Requirement: 205

Attempts on any step: No limits set

CS required at time of application: No

USCE Requirement: None

Cut-Off time since graduation: 4 years

Program offers couple match: No

Visas Sponsored or accepted: J1 visa and H1b visa

Icahn School of Medicine at Mount Sinai (Jamaica) Obstetrics and Gynecology Residency Program

Specialty: Obstetrics and Gynecology

Program name: Icahn School of Medicine at Mount Sinai (Jamaica) Program

Program code: 220-35-21-342

NRMP Code: 1489220C0

Program type: Community-based university

affiliated hospital
State: New York
Address: Queens Hospital Center
          82-68 164th St, Jamaica, NY 11432
Phone: (718) 883-4037
Fax: (718) 883-6129
Percentage of IMGs in the program: 80%
Minimum USMLE Step 1 Score Requirement:
No limits set
Minimum USMLE Step 2 Score Requirement:
No limits set
Attempts on any step: No limits set
CS required at time of application: Yes
including ECFMG certificate
USCE Requirement: None
Cut-Off time since graduation: No limits set
Program offers couple match: Yes
Visas Sponsored or accepted: J1 visa and H1b
visa

Nassau University Medical Center Obstetrics and Gynecology Residency Program

Specialty: Obstetrics and Gynecology
Program name: Nassau University Medical
Center Program
Program code: 220-35-31-174
State: New York

Address: Nassau University Medical Center
2201 Hempstead Trnpk, East Meadow, NY 11554
Phone: (516) 296-2830
Fax: (516) 572-3124
Percentage of IMGs in the program: 50%
Minimum USMLE Step 1 Score Requirement: No limits set
Minimum USMLE Step 2 Score Requirement: No limits set
Attempts on any step: No limits set
CS required at time of application: Yes including ECFMG certificate
USCE Requirement: None
Cut-Off time since graduation: 5 years
Program offers couple match: Yes
Visas Sponsored or accepted: J1 visa

Maimonides Medical Center Obstetrics and Gynecology Residency Program

Specialty: Obstetrics and Gynecology
Program name: Maimonides Medical Center Program
Program code: 220-35-31-192
NRMP Code: 1428220C0
Program type: Community-based
State: New York

Address: Maimonides Medical Center
4802 Tenth Ave, Brooklyn, NY 11219
Phone: (718) 283-6078
Fax: (718) 283-8468
Percentage of IMGs in the program: 60%
Minimum USMLE Step 1 Score Requirement:
No limits set
Minimum USMLE Step 2 Score Requirement:
No limits set
Attempts on any step: Must pass on first attempt
CS required at time of application: Yes including ECFMG certificate
USCE Requirement: None
Cut-Off time since graduation: No limits set
Program offers couple match: Yes
Visas Sponsored or accepted: J1 visa and H1b visa

New York Methodist Hospital Obstetrics and Gynecology Residency Program

Specialty: Obstetrics and Gynecology
Program name: New York Methodist Hospital Program
Program code: 220-35-31-339
NRMP Code: 1429220C0
Program type: Community-based university

affiliated hospital
State: New York
Address: New York Methodist Hospital
  506 Sixth St, Brooklyn, NY 11215
Phone: (718) 780-5213
Fax: (718) 780-3079
Percentage of IMGs in the program: 50%
Minimum USMLE Step 1 Score Requirement:
No limits set
Minimum USMLE Step 2 Score Requirement:
No limits set
Attempts on any step: No limits set
CS required at time of application: Yes
including ECFMG certificate
USCE Requirement: None
Cut-Off time since graduation: No limits set
Program offers couple match: Yes
Visas Sponsored or accepted: No visa

Rochester General Hospital Obstetrics and Gynecology Residency Program

Specialty: Obstetrics and Gynecology
Program name: Rochester General Hospital
Program
Program code: 220-35-31-343
NRMP Code: 1509220C0
Program type: Community-based university

affiliated hospital
State: New York
Address: Rochester General Hospital
1425 Portland Ave, Rochester, NY
14621-3095
Phone: (585) 922-4683
Fax: (585) 922-3606
Percentage of IMGs in the program: 95%
Minimum USMLE Step 1 Score Requirement:
No limits set
Minimum USMLE Step 2 Score Requirement:
No limits set
Attempts on any step: Must pass on first
attempt
CS required at time of application: Yes
including ECFMG certificate
USCE Requirement: None but preferred
Cut-Off time since graduation: No limits set
Program offers couple match: Yes
Visas Sponsored or accepted: J1 visa and H1b
visa

North Carolina

Vidant Medical Center/East Carolina University Obstetrics and Gynecology Residency Program

Specialty: Obstetrics and Gynecology
Program name: Vidant Medical Center/East Carolina University Program
Program code: 220-36-21-220
NRMP Code: 3057220C0
Program type: University-based
State: North Carolina
Address: Vidant Medical Center ECU
            600 Moye Blvd, Greenville, NC 27834
Phone: (252) 744-4669
Fax: (252) 744-5329
Percentage of IMGs in the program: 10%
Minimum USMLE Step 1 Score Requirement: No limits set
Minimum USMLE Step 2 Score Requirement: No limits set
Attempts on any step: No limits set
CS required at time of application: No
USCE Requirement: None
Cut-Off time since graduation: No limits set
Program offers couple match: Yes
Visas Sponsored or accepted: J1 visa

Wake Forest University School of Medicine Obstetrics and Gynecology Residency Program

Specialty: Obstetrics and Gynecology
Program name: Wake Forest University School of Medicine Program
Program code: 220-36-21-221
NRMP Code: 1537220C0
Program type: University-based
State: North Carolina
Address: Wake Forest Baptist Medical Center
Medical Center Blvd, Winston-Salem, NC 27157-1066
Phone: (336) 716-4615
Fax: (336) 716-6937
Percentage of IMGs in the program: 5%
Minimum USMLE Step 1 Score Requirement: No limits set
Minimum USMLE Step 2 Score Requirement: No limits set
Attempts on any step: No limits set
CS required at time of application: No
USCE Requirement: None
Cut-Off time since graduation: No limits set
Program offers couple match: Yes
Visas Sponsored or accepted: No visa

Ohio

TriHealth (Bethesda North and Good Samaritan Hospitals) Obstetrics and Gynecology Residency Program

Specialty: Obstetrics and Gynecology OB GYN Residency
Program name: TriHealth (Bethesda North and Good Samaritan Hospitals) Program
Program code: 220-38-11-228
NRMP Code: 1550220C0
Program type: Community-based
State: Ohio
Address: Good Samaritan Hospital
                375 Dixmyth Ave, Cincinnati, OH 45220
Phone: (513) 862-3400
Fax: (513) 221-5865
Percentage of IMGs in the program: 15%
Minimum USMLE Step 1 Score Requirement: 220
Minimum USMLE Step 2 Score Requirement: 220
Attempts on any step: Must pass maximum from the 2nd attempt

CS required at time of application: Yes including ECFMG certificate
USCE Requirement: Yes
Cut-Off time since graduation: 4 years
Program offers couple match: Yes
Visas Sponsored or accepted: No visa

Aultman Hospital/NEOMED Obstetrics and Gynecology Residency Program

Specialty: Obstetrics and Gynecology OB GYN Residency
Program name: Aultman Hospital/NEOMED Program
Program code: 220-38-21-226
NRMP Code: 1544220C0,
Program type: Community-based university affiliated hospital
State: Ohio
Address: Aultman Hospital
            2600 Sixth St SW, Canton, OH 44710-1799
Phone: (330) 994-1286
Fax: (330) 994-1296
Percentage of IMGs in the program: 25%
Minimum USMLE Step 1 Score Requirement: No limits set

Minimum USMLE Step 2 Score Requirement: No limits set
Attempts on any step: No limits set
CS required at time of application: No
USCE Requirement: None
Cut-Off time since graduation: No limits set
Program offers couple match: Yes
Visas Sponsored or accepted: J1 visa and H1b visa

Case Western Reserve University/University Hospitals Case Medical Center Obstetrics and Gynecology Residency Program

Specialty: Obstetrics and Gynecology OB GYN Residency
Program name: Case Western Reserve University/University Hospitals Case Medical Center Program
Program code: 220-38-21-230
State: Ohio
Address: University MacDonald Women's Hospital
11100 Euclid Ave, Cleveland, OH 44106
Phone: (216) 844-8551
Fax: (216) 201-4239
Percentage of IMGs in the program: 10%

Minimum USMLE Step 1 Score Requirement: No limits set

Minimum USMLE Step 2 Score Requirement: No limits set

Attempts on any step: Must pass on the first attempt

CS required at time of application: No

USCE Requirement: None

Cut-Off time since graduation: No limits set

Program offers couple match: Yes

Visas Sponsored or accepted: J1 visa

Case Western Reserve University (MetroHealth) Obstetrics and Gynecology Residency Program

Specialty: Obstetrics and Gynecology OB GYN Residency

Program name: Case Western Reserve University (MetroHealth) Program

Program code: 220-38-21-327

NRMP Code: 1553220P0, 1553220C0

Program type: University-based

State: Ohio

Address: MetroHealth Medical Center
          2500 MetroHealth Dr, Cleveland, OH 44109-1998

Phone: (216) 778-5539

Fax: (216) 778-8642

Percentage of IMGs in the program: 25%
Minimum USMLE Step 1 Score Requirement:
No limits set
Minimum USMLE Step 2 Score Requirement:
No limits set
Attempts on any step: No limits set
CS required at time of application: Yes
including ECFMG certificate
USCE Requirement: Yes, 1 month
Cut-Off time since graduation: No limits set
Program offers couple match: Yes
Visas Sponsored or accepted: J1 visa and H1b
visa

University of Toledo Obstetrics and Gynecology Residency Program

Specialty: Obstetrics and Gynecology OB GYN
Residency
Program name: University of Toledo Program
Program code: 220-38-22-237
NRMP Code: 1579220C0
Program type: University-based
State: Ohio
Address: University of Toledo Medical Center
        3120 Glendale Ave, Toledo, OH 43614-
5809
Phone: (419) 383-4590
Fax: (419) 383-3090

Percentage of IMGs in the program: 10%
Minimum USMLE Step 1 Score Requirement:
No limits set
Minimum USMLE Step 2 Score Requirement:
No limits set
Attempts on any step: Must pass on the first
attempt
CS required at time of application: No
USCE Requirement: None
Cut-Off time since graduation: 7 years
Program offers couple match: Yes
Visas Sponsored or accepted: J1 visa

Oklahoma

University of Oklahoma School of Community Medicine (Tulsa) Obstetrics and Gynecology Residency Program

Specialty: Obstetrics and Gynecology OB
GYN Residency
Program name: University of Oklahoma
School of Community Medicine (Tulsa)
Program
Program code: 220-39-21-240

State: Oklahoma
Address: University of Oklahoma College of Medicine Tulsa

       4502 E 41st St, Tulsa, OK 74135

Phone: (918) 660-8359
Fax: (918) 660-8355
Percentage of IMGs in the program: 10%
Minimum USMLE Step 1 Score Requirement: No limits set
Minimum USMLE Step 2 Score Requirement: No limits set
Attempts on any step: Must pass maximum from the 3rd attempt
CS required at time of application: Yes including ECFMG certificate
USCE Requirement: None
Cut-Off time since graduation: 5 years
Program offers couple match: Yes
Visas Sponsored or accepted: J1 visa and H1b visa

Pennsylvania

Lehigh Valley Health Network/University of South Florida College of Medicine Obstetrics and Gynecology Residency Program

Specialty: Obstetrics and Gynecology OB GYN Residency
Program name: Lehigh Valley Health Network/University of South Florida College of Medicine Program
Program code: 220-41-11-243
NRMP Code: 1601220C0
Program type: Community-based university affiliated hospital
State: Pennsylvania
Address: Lehigh Valley Health Network
          707 Hamilton St, Allentown, PA 18105-7017
Phone: (848) 862-3118
Fax: (848) 862-3102
Percentage of IMGs in the program: 10%
Minimum USMLE Step 1 Score Requirement: 210
Minimum USMLE Step 2 Score Requirement: 220
Attempts on any step: No limits set
CS required at time of application: Yes including ECFMG certificate
USCE Requirement: None

Cut-Off time since graduation: No limits set
Program offers couple match: Yes
Visas Sponsored or accepted: J1 visa and H1b visa

Main Line Health System/Lankenau Medical Center Obstetrics and Gynecology Residency Program

Specialty: Obstetrics and Gynecology OB GYN Residency
Program name: Main Line Health System/Lankenau Medical Center Program
Program code: 220-41-11-249
NRMP Code: 1632220C0
Program type: Community-based university affiliated hospital
State: Pennsylvania
Address: Lankenau Medical Center
        100 Lancaster Ave, Wynnewood, PA 19096
Phone: (484) 476-4650
Fax: (484) 476-2422
Percentage of IMGs in the program: 10%
Minimum USMLE Step 1 Score Requirement: No limits set
Minimum USMLE Step 2 Score Requirement: No limits set

Attempts on any step: Must pass on the first attempt
CS required at time of application: Yes including ECFMG certificate
USCE Requirement: Yes
Cut-Off time since graduation: 5 years
Program offers couple match: Yes
Visas Sponsored or accepted: J1 visa and H1b visa

Allegheny Health Network Medical Education Consortium (WPH) Obstetrics and Gynecology Residency Program

Specialty: Obstetrics and Gynecology OB GYN Residency
Program name: Allegheny Health Network Medical Education Consortium (WPH) Program
Program code: 220-41-11-261
NRMP Code: 1659220C0
Program type: Community-based university affiliated hospital
State: Pennsylvania
Address: Western Pennsylvania Hospital
4800 Friendship Ave, Pittsburgh, PA 15224
Phone: (412) 578-5587

Fax: (412) 578-4477
Percentage of IMGs in the program: 15%
Minimum USMLE Step 1 Score Requirement: 210
Minimum USMLE Step 2 Score Requirement: 210
Attempts on any step: No limits set
CS required at time of application: Yes including ECFMG certificate
USCE Requirement: None
Cut-Off time since graduation: No limits set
Program offers couple match: Yes
Visas Sponsored or accepted: J1 visa

Geisinger Health System Obstetrics and Gynecology Residency Program

Specialty: Obstetrics and Gynecology OB GYN Residency
Program name: Geisinger Health System Program
Program code: 220-41-12-245
State: Pennsylvania
Address: Geisinger Medical Center
        100 N Academy Ave, Danville, PA 17822-2920
Phone: (570) 271-5936
Fax: (570) 271-5819
Percentage of IMGs in the program: 15%

Minimum USMLE Step 1 Score Requirement: No limits set
Minimum USMLE Step 2 Score Requirement: No limits set
Attempts on any step: Must pass on the first attempt
CS required at time of application: Yes including ECFMG certificate
USCE Requirement: None
Cut-Off time since graduation: 5 years
Program offers couple match: Yes
Visas Sponsored or accepted: J1 visa

Penn State Milton S Hershey Medical Center Obstetrics and Gynecology Residency Program

Specialty: Obstetrics and Gynecology OB GYN Residency
Program name: Penn State Milton S Hershey Medical Center Program
Program code: 220-41-21-246
NRMP Code: 1617220C0
Program type: University-based
State: Pennsylvania
Address: Penn State Hershey Medical Center
500 University Dr, Hershey, PA 17033-0850
Phone: (717) 531-5394

Fax: (717) 531-0066
Percentage of IMGs in the program: 5%
Minimum USMLE Step 1 Score Requirement:
No limits set
Minimum USMLE Step 2 Score Requirement:
No limits set
Attempts on any step: No limits set
CS required at time of application: No
USCE Requirement: None
Cut-Off time since graduation: No limits set
Program offers couple match: Yes
Visas Sponsored or accepted: J1 visa

Albert Einstein Healthcare Network Obstetrics and Gynecology Residency Program

Specialty: Obstetrics and Gynecology OB GYN
Residency
Program name: Albert Einstein Healthcare
Network Program
Program code: 220-41-21-247
NRMP Code: 1631220C0
Program type: Community-based
State: Pennsylvania
Address: Albert Einstein Medical Center
        5501 Old York Rd, Philadelphia, PA
19141-3098
Phone: (215) 456-8261
Fax: (215) 456-4958

Percentage of IMGs in the program: 50%
Minimum USMLE Step 1 Score Requirement: 220
Minimum USMLE Step 2 Score Requirement: 220
Attempts on any step: No limits set
CS required at time of application: Yes including ECFMG certificate
USCE Requirement: None
Cut-Off time since graduation: No limits set
Program offers couple match: Yes
Visas Sponsored or accepted: J1 visa and H1b visa

Drexel University College of Medicine/Hahnemann University Hospital Obstetrics and Gynecology Residency Program

Specialty: Obstetrics and Gynecology OB GYN Residency
Program name: Drexel University College of Medicine/Hahnemann University Hospital Program
Program code: 220-41-21-250
NRMP Code: 1849220C0
Program type: University-based
State: Pennsylvania

Address: Drexel University College of Medicine
245 N 15th St, Philadelphia, PA
19102-1192
Phone: (215) 762-8220
Fax: (215) 762-1470
Percentage of IMGs in the program: 40%
Minimum USMLE Step 1 Score Requirement:
No limits set
Minimum USMLE Step 2 Score Requirement:
No limits set
Attempts on any step: No limits set
CS required at time of application: Yes
including ECFMG certificate
USCE Requirement: None
Cut-Off time since graduation: 4 years
Program offers couple match: Yes
Visas Sponsored or accepted: J1 visa

Temple University Hospital Obstetrics and Gynecology Residency Program

Specialty: Obstetrics and Gynecology OB GYN
Residency
Program name: Temple University Hospital
Program
Program code: 220-41-21-254
State: Pennsylvania

Address: Temple University Hospital
3401 N Broad St, Philadelphia, PA 19140
Phone: (215) 707-3187
Fax: (215) 707-1387
Percentage of IMGs in the program: 0% (Occasionally 1 match)
Minimum USMLE Step 1 Score Requirement: No limits set
Minimum USMLE Step 2 Score Requirement: No limits set
Attempts on any step: No limits set
CS required at time of application: Yes including ECFMG certificate
USCE Requirement: None
Cut-Off time since graduation: 5 years
Program offers couple match: No
Visas Sponsored or accepted: J1 visa and H1b visa

Crozer-Chester Medical Center Obstetrics and Gynecology Residency Program

Specialty: Obstetrics and Gynecology OB GYN Residency
Program name: Crozer-Chester Medical Center Program

Program code: 220-41-21-367
NRMP Code: 3185220C0
Program type: Community-based university affiliated hospital
State: Pennsylvania
Address: Crozer-Chester Medical Center
          One Medical Center Blvd, Upland, PA 19013
Phone: (610) 447-7612
Fax: (610) 447-7615
Percentage of IMGs in the program: 60%
Minimum USMLE Step 1 Score Requirement: No limits set
Minimum USMLE Step 2 Score Requirement: No limits set
Attempts on any step: No limits set
CS required at time of application: No
USCE Requirement: None
Cut-Off time since graduation: No limits set
Program offers couple match: No
Visas Sponsored or accepted: J1 visa and H1b visa

St Luke's Hospital Obstetrics and Gynecology Residency Program

Specialty: Obstetrics and Gynecology OB GYN Residency
Program name: St Luke's Hospital Program
Program code: 220-41-31-244

NRMP Code: 1605220C0
Program type: Community-based university affiliated hospital
State: Pennsylvania
Address: St Luke's University Health Network
         801 Ostrum St, Bethlehem, PA 18015
Phone: (484) 526-4670
Fax: (484) 526-2381
Percentage of IMGs in the program: 40%
Minimum USMLE Step 1 Score Requirement: 220
Minimum USMLE Step 2 Score Requirement: 220
Attempts on any step: No limits set
CS required at time of application: No
USCE Requirement: None
Cut-Off time since graduation: No limits set
Program offers couple match: No
Visas Sponsored or accepted: J1 visa and H1b visa

South Carolina

Palmetto Health/University of South Carolina School of Medicine Obstetrics and Gynecology Residency Program

Specialty: Obstetrics and Gynecology
Program name: Palmetto Health/University of South Carolina School of Medicine Program
Program code: 220-45-11-271
State: South Carolina
Address: Palmetto Health Richland Hospital, Suite 208,
Two Medical Park, Columbia, SC 29203
Phone: (803) 545-5702
Fax: (803) 434-4699
Percentage of IMGs in the program: 10%
Minimum USMLE Step 1 Score Requirement: No limits set
Minimum USMLE Step 2 Score Requirement: No limits set
Attempts on any step: No limits set
CS required at time of application: Yes including ECFMG certificate
USCE Requirement: None
Cut-Off time since graduation: 5 years
Program offers couple match: Yes
Visas Sponsored or accepted: No visa

Tennessee

University of Tennessee College of Medicine at Chattanooga Obstetrics and Gynecology Residency Program

Specialty: Obstetrics and Gynecology OB GYN Residency
Program name: University of Tennessee College of Medicine at Chattanooga Program
Program code: 220-47-21-274
NRMP Code: 1689220C0
Program type: University-based
State: Tennessee
Address: University of Tennessee College of Medicine-Chattanooga
979 E Third St, Chattanooga, TN 37403
Phone: (423) 778-7515
Fax: (423) 778-7522
Percentage of IMGs in the program: 20%
Minimum USMLE Step 1 Score Requirement: No limits set
Minimum USMLE Step 2 Score Requirement: No limits set
Attempts on any step: Must pass on the first attempt
CS required at time of application: Yes including ECFMG certificate

USCE Requirement: None
Cut-Off time since graduation: No limits set
Program offers couple match: Yes
Visas Sponsored or accepted: J1 visa

University of Tennessee Obstetrics and Gynecology Residency Program

Specialty: Obstetrics and Gynecology OB GYN Residency
Program name: University of Tennessee Program
Program code: 220-47-21-276
NRMP Code: 1844220C0
Program type: University-based
State: Tennessee
Address: University of Tennessee Health Science Center
        853 Jefferson Ave, Memphis, TN 38163
Phone: (901) 448-4795
Fax: (901) 448-7075
Percentage of IMGs in the program: 15%
Minimum USMLE Step 1 Score Requirement: No limits set
Minimum USMLE Step 2 Score Requirement: No limits set
Attempts on any step: No limits set
CS required at time of application: No
USCE Requirement: None

Cut-Off time since graduation: 5 years unless clinically active for at least 2 years during the last 7 years
Program offers couple match: Yes
Visas Sponsored or accepted: J1 visa

Vanderbilt University Obstetrics and Gynecology Residency Program

Specialty: Obstetrics and Gynecology OB GYN Residency
Program name: Vanderbilt University Program
Program code: 220-47-21-278
NRMP Code: 1702220C0
Program type: University-based
State: Tennessee
Address: Vanderbilt University Medical Center
1611 21st Ave S, Nashville, TN 37232-2521
Phone: (615) 343-8801
Fax: (615) 343-8806
Percentage of IMGs in the program: 10%
Minimum USMLE Step 1 Score Requirement: 215
Minimum USMLE Step 2 Score Requirement: 215
Attempts on any step: No limits set
CS required at time of application: Yes including ECFMG certificate
USCE Requirement: Yes

Cut-Off time since graduation: 5 years
Program offers couple match: Yes
Visas Sponsored or accepted: J1 visa

East Tennessee State University Obstetrics and Gynecology Residency Program

Specialty: Obstetrics and Gynecology OB GYN Residency
Program name: East Tennessee State University Program
Program code: 220-47-21-341
NRMP Code: 2066220C0
Program type: University-based
State: Tennessee
Address: ETSU James H Quillen College of Medicine
          PO Box 70569, Johnson City, TN 37614
Phone: (423) 439-6262
Fax: (423) 439-6766
Percentage of IMGs in the program: 15%
Minimum USMLE Step 1 Score Requirement: 220
Minimum USMLE Step 2 Score Requirement: 220
Attempts on any step: Must pass maximum on the 2nd attempt

CS required at time of application: Yes including ECFMG certificate
USCE Requirement: 12 months
Cut-Off time since graduation: 3 years
Program offers couple match: Yes
Visas Sponsored or accepted: J1 visa

Texas

University of Texas RGV (DHR) Obstetrics and Gynecology Residency Program

Specialty: Obstetrics and Gynecology OB GYN Residency
Program name: University of Texas RGV (DHR) Program
Program code: 220-48-00-361
State: Texas
Address: University of Texas Rio Grande Valley - Doctors Hospital at Renaissance
2821 Michaelangelo Dr, Edinburg, TX 78539
Phone: (956) 362-3594
Fax: (956) 362-3598
Percentage of IMGs in the program: 10%

Minimum USMLE Step 1 Score Requirement: No limits set
Minimum USMLE Step 2 Score Requirement: No limits set
Attempts on any step: No limits set
CS required at time of application: Yes including ECFMG certificate
USCE Requirement: None
Cut-Off time since graduation: No limits set
Program offers couple match: Yes
Visas Sponsored or accepted: J1 visa

Texas Tech University Health Sciences Center Paul L Foster School of Medicine Obstetrics and Gynecology Residency Program

Specialty: Obstetrics and Gynecology OB GYN Residency
Program name: Texas Tech University Health Sciences Center Paul L Foster School of Medicine Program
Program code: 220-48-11-315
NRMP Code: 1710220C0
Program type: University-based
State: Texas
Address: Texas Tech University HSC Paul L Foster School of Medicine
          4800 Alberta Ave, El Paso, TX 79905
Phone: (915) 215-5020

Fax: (915) 545-0901
Percentage of IMGs in the program: 5%
Minimum USMLE Step 1 Score Requirement: 210
Minimum USMLE Step 2 Score Requirement: 210
Attempts on any step: Must pass on the first attempt
CS required at time of application: Yes including ECFMG certificate
USCE Requirement: None
Cut-Off time since graduation: No limits set
Program offers couple match: Yes
Visas Sponsored or accepted: No visa

University of Texas Medical Branch Hospitals Obstetrics and Gynecology Residency Program

Specialty: Obstetrics and Gynecology OB GYN Residency
Program name: University of Texas Medical Branch Hospitals Program
Program code: 220-48-21-285
NRMP Code: 1714220C0
Program type: University-based
State: Texas
Address: University of Texas Med Branch Hospitals

301 University Blvd, Galveston, TX 77555-0587
Phone: (409) 772-2999
Fax: (409) 772-5803
Percentage of IMGs in the program: 10%
Minimum USMLE Step 1 Score Requirement: No limits set
Minimum USMLE Step 2 Score Requirement: No limits set
Attempts on any step: Must pass maximum from the 3rd attempt
CS required at time of application: No
USCE Requirement: 12 months
Cut-Off time since graduation: 3 years
Program offers couple match: Yes
Visas Sponsored or accepted: J1 visa

University of Texas Health Science Center at Houston (Memorial Hermann Hospital) Obstetrics and Gynecology Residency Program

Specialty: Obstetrics and Gynecology OB GYN Residency
Program name: University of Texas Health Science Center at Houston (Memorial Hermann Hospital) Program
Program code: 220-48-21-289
NRMP Code: 2923220C0
Program type: University-based

State: Texas
Address: University of Texas Medical School
Houston
      6431 Fannin St, Houston, TX 77030
Phone: (713) 500-6397
Fax: (713) 500-0798
Percentage of IMGs in the program: 10%
Minimum USMLE Step 1 Score Requirement:
No limits set
Minimum USMLE Step 2 Score Requirement:
No limits set
Attempts on any step: Must pass maximum on
the 3rd attempt
CS required at time of application: Yes
including ECFMG certificate
USCE Requirement: None
Cut-Off time since graduation: No limits set
Program offers couple match: Yes
Visas Sponsored or accepted: J1 visa

Texas Tech University (Lubbock) Obstetrics and Gynecology Residency Program

Specialty: Obstetrics and Gynecology OB GYN
Residency
Program name: Texas Tech University
(Lubbock) Program
Program code: 220-48-21-290
NRMP Code: 2973220C0

Program type: Community-based university affiliated hospital
State: Texas
Address: Texas Tech University HSC Lubbock
3601 4th St, Lubbock, TX 79430
Phone: (806) 743-3039
Fax: (806) 743-2174
Percentage of IMGs in the program: 40%
Minimum USMLE Step 1 Score Requirement: No limits set
Minimum USMLE Step 2 Score Requirement: No limits set
Attempts on any step: Must pass maximum on the 3rd attempt
CS required at time of application: Yes including ECFMG certificate
USCE Requirement: None
Cut-Off time since graduation: No limits set
Program offers couple match: Yes
Visas Sponsored or accepted: J1 visa

Texas Tech University (Permian Basin) Obstetrics and Gynecology Residency Program

Specialty: Obstetrics and Gynecology OB GYN Residency
Program name: Texas Tech University (Permian Basin) Program

Program code: 220-48-21-331
NRMP Code: 3124220C0
Program type: University-based
State: Texas
Address: Texas Tech University HSC Odessa
          701 W 5th St, Odessa, TX 79763-4362
Phone: (432) 703-5050
Fax: (432) 335-5240
Percentage of IMGs in the program: 10%
Minimum USMLE Step 1 Score Requirement:
No limits set
Minimum USMLE Step 2 Score Requirement:
No limits set
Attempts on any step: Must pass maximum on
the 3rd attempt
CS required at time of application: Yes
including ECFMG certificate
USCE Requirement: Yes
Cut-Off time since graduation: No limits set
Program offers couple match: Yes
Visas Sponsored or accepted: J1 visa

University of Texas Health Science
Center at Houston (Lyndon B
Johnson General Hospital)
Obstetrics and Gynecology
Residency Program

Specialty: Obstetrics and Gynecology OB GYN Residency
Program name: University of Texas Health Science Center at Houston (Lyndon B Johnson General Hospital) Program
Program code: 220-48-21-334
NRMP Code: 2923220C1
Program type: University-based
State: Texas
Address: Lyndon B Johnson General Hospital
5656 Kelley St, Houston, TX 77026
Phone: (713) 566-5735
Fax: (713) 566-4521
Percentage of IMGs in the program: 15%
Minimum USMLE Step 1 Score Requirement: No limits set
Minimum USMLE Step 2 Score Requirement: No limits set
Attempts on any step: Must pass maximum on the 3rd attempt
CS required at time of application: Yes including ECFMG certificate
USCE Requirement: None
Cut-Off time since graduation: No limits set
Program offers couple match: Yes
Visas Sponsored or accepted: J1 visa

Methodist Health System Dallas Obstetrics and Gynecology Residency Program

Specialty: Obstetrics and Gynecology OB GYN Residency
Program name: Methodist Health System Dallas Program
Program code: 220-48-31-281
NRMP Code: 1707220C0
Program type: Community-based
State: Texas
Address: Methodist Health System Dallas
1441 N Beckley Ave, Dallas, TX 75203
Phone: (214) 947-2331
Fax: (214) 947-2361
Percentage of IMGs in the program: 10%
Minimum USMLE Step 1 Score Requirement: 210
Minimum USMLE Step 2 Score Requirement: 210
Attempts on any step: Must pass on the first attempt
CS required at time of application: Yes including ECFMG certificate
USCE Requirement: None
Cut-Off time since graduation: 2 years
Program offers couple match: Yes
Visas Sponsored or accepted: No visa

Methodist Hospital (Houston) Obstetrics and Gynecology Residency Program

Specialty: Obstetrics and Gynecology OB GYN Residency
Program name: Methodist Hospital (Houston) Program
Program code: 220-48-31-288
NRMP Code: 1167220C0
Program type: Community-based
State: Texas
Address: Houston Methodist Hospital
1401 St Joseph Pkwy, Houston, TX 77002
Phone: (713) 756-8374
Fax: (713) 657-7191
Percentage of IMGs in the program: 5%
Minimum USMLE Step 1 Score Requirement: 220
Minimum USMLE Step 2 Score Requirement: 230
Attempts on any step: Must pass maximum from the 2nd attempt
CS required at time of application: No
USCE Requirement: None
Cut-Off time since graduation: 3 years
Program offers couple match: Yes
Visas Sponsored or accepted: J1 visa and H1b visa

Virginia

Inova Fairfax Medical Campus Obstetrics and Gynecology Residency Program

Specialty: Obstetrics and Gynecology
Program name: Inova Fairfax Medical Campus Program
Program code: 220-51-00-301
State: Virginia
Address: Women's & Children's Hospital
3300 Gallows Rd, Falls Church, VA 22042
Phone: (703) 776-2745
Fax: (866) 291-4915
Percentage of IMGs in the program: 40%
Minimum USMLE Step 1 Score Requirement: No limits set
Minimum USMLE Step 2 Score Requirement: No limits set

Attempts on any step: Must pass on first attempt
CS required at time of application: Yes
USCE Requirement: None
Cut-Off time since graduation: 5 years preferred
Program offers couple match: Yes
Visas Sponsored or accepted: J1 visa and H1b visa

Riverside Regional Medical Center Obstetrics and Gynecology Residency Program

Specialty: Obstetrics and Gynecology
Program name: Riverside Regional Medical Center Program
Program code: 220-51-11-297
NRMP Code: 1739220C0
Program type: Community-based
State: Virginia
Address: Riverside Regional Medical Center
500 J Clyde Morris Blvd, Newport News, VA 23601
Phone: (757) 594-4737
Fax: (757) 594-3184
Percentage of IMGs in the program: 40%
Minimum USMLE Step 1 Score Requirement: No limits set

Minimum USMLE Step 2 Score Requirement: No limits set

Attempts on any step: No limits set

CS required at time of application: Yes including ECFMG certificate

USCE Requirement: Yes 2 different rotations 1 month each

Cut-Off time since graduation: No limits set but must have any clinical experience in the last 2 years

Program offers couple match: Yes

Visas Sponsored or accepted: J1 visa

Eastern Virginia Medical School Obstetrics and Gynecology Residency Program

Specialty: Obstetrics and Gynecology

Program name: Eastern Virginia Medical School Program

Program code: 220-51-21-298

NRMP Code: 2980220C0

Program type: Community-based

State: Virginia

Address: Eastern Virginia Medical School
825 Fairfax Ave, Norfolk, VA 23507

Phone: (757) 446-7470

Fax: (757) 446-7464

Percentage of IMGs in the program: 15%

Minimum USMLE Step 1 Score Requirement: No limits set
Minimum USMLE Step 2 Score Requirement: No limits set
Attempts on any step: Must pass on first attempt
CS required at time of application: Yes including ECFMG certificate
USCE Requirement: None
Cut-Off time since graduation: 8 years
Program offers couple match: Yes
Visas Sponsored or accepted: J1 visa

West Virginia

Charleston Area Medical Center/West Virginia University (Charleston Division) Obstetrics and Gynecology Residency Program

Specialty: Obstetrics and Gynecology
Program name: Charleston Area Medical Center/West Virginia University (Charleston Division) Program
Program code: 220-55-11-303
NRMP Code: 1902220C0
Program type: Community-based university affiliated hospital

State: West Virginia
Address: West Virginia University Charleston Division

   830 Pennsylvania Ave, Charleston, WV 25302
Phone: (304) 388-1515
Fax: (304) 388-1586
Percentage of IMGs in the program: 8% (Variable)
Minimum USMLE Step 1 Score Requirement: 200
Minimum USMLE Step 2 Score Requirement: 205
Attempts on any step: Must pass on first attempt
CS required at time of application: No
USCE Requirement: None
Cut-Off time since graduation: No limits set
Program offers couple match: Yes
Visas Sponsored or accepted: J1 visa

Marshall University School of Medicine Obstetrics and Gynecology Residency Program

Specialty: Obstetrics and Gynecology
Program name: Marshall University School of Medicine Program
Program code: 220-55-21-344

NRMP Code: 3066220C0
Program type: Community-based university affiliated hospital
State: West Virginia
Address: Marshall University School of Medicine
1600 Medical Center Dr, Huntington, WV 25701-3655
Phone: (304) 691-1454   Ext: 1454
Fax: (304) 691-1453
Percentage of IMGs in the program: 20%
Minimum USMLE Step 1 Score Requirement: 200 (188 previously)
Minimum USMLE Step 2 Score Requirement: 205 (196 previously)
Attempts on any step: No limits set
CS required at time of application: Yes
USCE Requirement: None
Cut-Off time since graduation: No limits set
Program offers couple match: Yes
Visas Sponsored or accepted: J1 visa

Wisconsin

Aurora Health Care Obstetrics and Gynecology Residency Program

Specialty: Obstetrics and Gynecology
Program name: Aurora Health Care Program
Program code: 220-56-12-308
NRMP Code: 1787220C0
Program type: Community-based
State: Wisconsin
Address: Aurora Sinai Medical Center
              945 N 12th St, Milwaukee, WI 53201-0342
Phone: (414) 219-5725
Fax: (414) 219-5611
Percentage of IMGs in the program: 10%
Minimum USMLE Step 1 Score Requirement: No limits set
Minimum USMLE Step 2 Score Requirement: No limits set
Attempts on any step: Must pass on first attempt
CS required at time of application: Yes including ECFMG certificate
USCE Requirement: Yes
Cut-Off time since graduation: 2 years
Program offers couple match: Yes
Visas Sponsored or accepted: No visa

Please take 1 minute to write a review and rate our book on Amazon. We wish you a successful match. Thank you for buying our book.

If you have any questions please email us at applicantguide@yahoo.com

IMG Guide
&
Applicant Guide

www.imgguide.com
www.applicantguide.com